The Most Important
60 Days of Your Pregnancy

The Most Important
60 Days of Your Pregnancy

Prevent Your Child from Developing Diabetes and Obesity Later in Life

Dr. Pierre Dukan

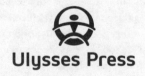

Ulysses Press

Published in the United States by:
Ulysses Press
P.O. Box 3440
Berkeley, CA 94703
www.ulyssespress.com

ISBN: 978-1-61243-729-3
Library of Congress Control Number 2017938175

Printed in Canada by Marquis Book Printing
10 9 8 7 6 5 4 3 2 1

Acquisitions: Casie Vogel
Managing editor: Claire Chun
Editor: Renee Rutledge
Proofreader: Shayna Keyles
Indexer: Sayre Van Young
Front cover design: what!design @ whatweb.com
Cover photos: © Africa Studio/shutterstock.com
Interior design: Jake Flaherty

Distributed by Publishers Group West

NOTE TO READERS: This book has been written and published strictly for informational and educational purposes only. It is not intended to serve as medical advice or to be any form of medical treatment. You should always consult your physician before altering or changing any aspect of your medical treatment and/or undertaking a diet regimen, including the guidelines as described in this book. Do not stop or change any prescription medications without the guidance and advice of your physician. Any use of the information in this book is made on the reader's good judgment after consulting with his or her physician and is the reader's sole responsibility. This book is not intended to diagnose or treat any medical condition and is not a substitute for a physician.

This book is independently authored and published and no sponsorship or endorsement of this book by, and no affiliation with, any trademarked brands or other products mentioned within is claimed or suggested. All trademarks that appear in this book belong to their respective owners and are used here for informational purposes only. The author and publishers encourage readers to patronize the quality brands mentioned in this book.

Contents

Introduction

I've worked as a general practitioner for over 40 years and have seen many diet programs come and go. Now, after years of research, I've developed new nutritional guidelines that will produce real and meaningful results. It is my deepest hope that the information found in this book will help stop the spread of excess weight, obesity, and diabetes—conditions that are at epidemic levels.

My goal is to draw attention to a fact that is all too often covered up or ignored. Humanity today and the generations that will follow face a grave threat. Global statistics show that this danger has now been in our midst for two generations. In the post-war years, people that were considered overweight numbered in the hundreds of millions; since then, the number has skyrocketed to two billion.

The crisis of excess weight, obesity, and diabetes has long been treated as a somewhat trivial issue. This has been due, at times, to short-sightedness, and at other times, to complicity. But we now know that weight problems impair or adversely affect the life and well-being of one out of two adults in the West, directly or indirectly leading to the deaths of 75 million people.

The Most Important 60 Days

In this book, I pay close attention to nutrition in the final six months of pregnancy, with a special focus on the fourth and fifth months—60 important days—wherein the baby's pancreas develops and begins secreting insulin. During this time, when she is influenced by maternal hormones and senses instinctively what might pose a risk to her baby, a pregnant woman is capable of choosing to change her status from "consumer" to "mother."

The information I've laid out in this book appeals to a pregnant woman's common sense and maternal instincts and allows her to do the following:

- Understand that what she eats during pregnancy can radically change the life of her child, and make decisions accordingly.

- Understand and accept that many of the foods she now consumes are tolerable for her but may not be tolerable to her unborn child.

In response to my recommendation to follow this plan, one of my patients responded with a wonderful crystallization of my thoughts: "Basically," she said, "you're asking me to eat for six months the way people ate in my grandmother's time."

It's well worth considering that in your grandmother's time, the abundance of mass-produced breads and industrially processed foods so popular today were not available. By processed, I mean industrially produced—refined, altered, and stripped of their fiber. Specifically, I mean white sugar extracted from red beets, and genetically modified white flour; both are nutritional wastelands.

My goal can be boiled down to this: I want to convince you to eat the way people ate only two generations ago. And I particularly want you to do so during the fourth and fifth months of your pregnancy—the most decisive months for the development of the pancreas of the child you're carrying.

How this Program Began

I began my medical studies in a period when, to the dismay of health and medical institutions, the number of overweight persons in France reached one million. At the end of my 10 years of medical studies, I became extremely frustrated as I discovered that the dogma focused on calories was proving very ineffective for those who want to lose weight.

I watched the crisis turn into an epidemic. The numbers continued to rise with dizzying speed: 27 million French citizens were overweight. The phenomenon seemed universal, borderless. As I watched the developments closely, I was struck by a number of points that I observed but couldn't yet understand.

1. In the space of 30 years, from 1970 to 2000, the average birth weight of infants in the West underwent a startling increase.

In 1970, the average birth weight was 6.6 pounds; by 2000, the number had risen to 7.7 pounds. This neared the limit for what was considered overweight. Today, however, 7.7 pounds is the norm, and only an infant of 8.8 pounds or more is considered a big baby.

What explains this significant increase in birth weight? We know that the fetus lives a completely passive life, depending solely on food from the mother. Scientifically and logically, then, the only possible explanation is a substantial change in maternal nutrition, on a global scale. Pregnant women are actually eating less than they did in the past; but, they are eating differently. Along with the rest of the population, their diet has been overtaken by an entirely new category of foods. This category consists of foods that have been industrially transformed, processed, concentrated, and refined, becoming what I will call invasive carbohydrates. The term is meant to emphasize the lightning speed with which these carbohydrates are digested and assimilated.

2. The overweight population has grown with alarming speed.

After starting slowly in the 1950s, the problem accelerated drastically in the 1970s, affecting one quarter of the world's population in just 20 years. In my mind, there was no way such a progression could be explained by overeating and sedentary lifestyles alone.

3. Type 2 diabetes began to make an appearance in children and adolescents, a condition that previously affected only adults.

This aberrant phenomenon is strongest in developing countries, where food cultures have changed radically. Diabetes rates for children in China are four times higher than diabetes rates for children in the US. These rates mirror a sharp rise in obesity, which is affecting children at a younger and younger age. Who do we blame for the fact that one in six children is obese, or for the fact that the signs of this obesity can already be detected at the age of two or three? Accusing children at that age of overconsumption or inactivity would be nonsensical.

4. The prevalence of gestational diabetes has increased.

Gestational diabetes is diabetes that appears during a pregnancy, typically during the last trimester. We know that hormones secreted naturally by the placenta make insulin less effective; this is known as insulin resistance. This forces the pancreas to secrete more insulin for protection. The exertion can exhaust the pancreas and induce temporary diabetes.

In evolutionary terms, this phenomenon, related to fat storage, probably represented an advantage, offering protection for pregnancy during times of scarcity. But the flood of invasive and highly processed sugars in the modern diet (and therefore in the diet of pregnant women) exceeds the abilities of the pancreas to control blood sugar levels.

This is evidenced by the fact that the number of women affected by gestational diabetes varies according to country and culture. For instance, the prevalence of the condition in France today ranges from 6 to 10 percent; in the US, however, where sugar is consumed in higher proportions, it can be as high as 18 percent. The many consequences of gestational diabetes include the risk of the child being born larger than is optimal, being more likely to become obese at the start of adulthood, and more easily developing glucose intolerance, which can develop into diabetes.

5. The concept of "diabesity"—a combination of diabetes and obesity—emerged.

These two conditions were long considered distinct, until a common cause was finally discovered: extra insulin produced by the pancreas to deal with the onslaught of invasive sugars.

I found these five points perplexing. They seemed to be linked, but the relation between them was a mystery. This mystery troubled me for a long time. I needed to find the connection between them. The opportunity came when I transferred my patients' files to a digital format. The change made it possible to compare their data more extensively and in much greater detail.

Exploring the new database, I discovered a link between my patients' dietary choices during pregnancy and the birth weight of their children. For some long-term patients, there was also information on the evolution of their children's diet and health to adolescence. My findings contained nothing absolute, but they were enough to focus my attention on pregnancy.

Introducing the Program

I formed the suspicion that not all calories are equal and that what really matters is the type of calorie, or the nutrient it carries. In talking with my patients, I found that the vast majority gain weight from eating too many invasive carbohydrates.

Over time, I built a diet that eliminates these sugars during a relatively brief period of weight loss. The results of this method confirmed that excess weight is a condition that could be mastered by those who have the motivation to give up these sugars during the weight-loss phase. I went on to share this method in my book, *The Dukan Diet*, which reached readers all over the world. Reaching millions of readers is quite a success, but only readers that have what I call DLW, Determination to Lose Weight, will succeed in shedding pounds, and often, in maintaining their new weight.

But there are many whose motivation hasn't reached this level, who don't have a strong relationship with a doctor, and who suffer from a wealth of misinformation. In the fight against excess weight, these individuals are simply outmatched. Why is it so hard for them?

People gain weight despite their aversion to the extra pounds because they can't resist foods that make them overweight. This is partly because the food industry is built around sugar, white flour, and processed foods made with these products. From birth to the age of 50, people are bombarded with pressure to eat processed foods that cause them to gain weight.

The food industry alone does not benefit from this; the pharmaceutical industry also profits from an overweight population. From the age of 50 on, people try to protect their health with extremely expensive drugs for weight-related diseases.

It's hard for most people to grasp the enormous power of the major food producers, or the extent of their ties to the medical community and the media. All of this contributes to the epidemic that we see today, one that can be combated if expectant mothers have the right tools and knowledge about what foods to eat during the most important 60 days of pregnancy. That is my aim in this writing this book.

It's important to note that this information has its roots firmly embedded in an immense body of collective scientific work. I took many scientific studies, surveys, research projects, and observations from every continent into account to ensure that the information and nutritional plan in this book is sound.

Chapter 1 focuses on the enemies: excess weight, obesity, and diabetes. It is essential to recognize the seriousness of these problems. This chapter sets the stage for the rest of the book, which will give you the means to avoid these risks for your unborn child over the course of your pregnancy.

All too often we talk about weight problems without discussing the reasons for them. Thus, **Chapter 2** focuses on the deep and hidden causes of these conditions: their physical, mental, and social components.

Chapter 3 is devoted to information about the cycle of sugar intake and insulin release, including a discussion on the growing body of knowledge available to the public on the dangers of this cycle.

Chapter 4 focuses on how the pancreas appears during the pregnancy and develops within your baby's abdomen. I have already said that overeating and a sedentary lifestyle alone could never lead to an epidemic of this proportion. In my view, the scope of the crisis is related to the arrival of a generation of newborns whose pancreas has been left vulnerable, which leads to an exponential increase in the number of individuals affected. To understand my plan and to be able to follow it, you will need to understand how this unique organ functions and develops, including the centerpiece of my plan, the science of epigenetics.

Chapter 5 offers guidance on how to practice the plan, including lists of foods to avoid and eat freely during three distinct phases of your pregnancy, with a special emphasis on the most important 60 days—months four and five. You'll be surprised how simple the measures are. In no time at all, you'll be speeding toward victory. Not a single dietary measure in this plan will disadvantage you or cause you or your unborn child any risk. Each step will be nothing but beneficial to the health of you both.

Chapter 1

The Risks and Dangers of Excess Weight, Obesity, and Diabetes

The weight crisis has progressed with incredible speed and generated untold harm. We can't go on excusing it as a symptom of *joie de vivre*, or a happy and carefree lifestyle. Excess weight has become a terribly efficient killer; indeed, it's the leading health risk threatening us today.

Excess weight is a recent problem. Before 1944, only a slim portion of the population was affected. Being heavy, or even obese, was seen as a visible sign of wealth and power. It meant prominence, in the most literal sense of the word.

In prewar France, an estimated 100,000 people were overweight or obese. By 1960, there were over a million. In 2009, 27 million people were overweight with a BMI between 25 and 30; seven million of these were obese with a BMI above 30. The lifespan of the obese was *nine years* shorter. And, in fact, France was more successful than most countries at resisting the epidemic. If France had the same proportion of overweight people as the US did at the time, obesity numbers would be twice what they are now.

What explains this phenomenon? How is it related to historical context, and how has it progressed? The usual explanation for the weight crisis is simple: It is caused by caloric intake exceeding energy expenditure. Unfortunately, the answer adds nothing to our understanding. It offers us the *how* of the weight crisis, but not the *why*.

So now, let's ask why.

The goal of this book is to show—in a demonstrable, scientific way—that if you are nurturing an unborn child in your womb, *you have the power to take decisive action for your child's future weight.* And if all the mothers in the world shared that understanding and were aware of the simple measures that followed from it, it would be possible to stop the progression of the weight crisis—even to reverse it.

That claim might seem bold, even utopic. How could we even conceive of stopping the scourge so easily, one that has already caused tens of millions of deaths around the world? No country on Earth has been able to do so.

The objections are understandable. All I ask is that you read on. I've spent three full years working on this project, and I haven't worked alone. I've spoken with dozens of committed scientists who specialize in this area, and analyzed thousands of studies on the subject.

There's no disputing the fact that from the time our species came into being some 200,000 years ago up to the middle of the last century, expectant mothers nourished their unborn children with a stable, nutritious diet, despite cultural and geographic variations.

Yet, since the middle of the last century, this diet has collapsed. That collapse has been simultaneous with the weight crisis. The imbalance that now exists is due to the industrialization of human food production. Food has become merchandise. As such, it is subject to the usual demands of cost reduction and productivity. The priority is profit, with no regard for the nutritional consequences.

The industries dependent on the intensive production of sugar, flour, and their derivatives are making their fortunes by making us fat, from birth to middle age. Then, in our golden years, the pharmaceutical industry profits by selling us treatments for the health problems caused by excess weight.

Our societies are governed by economics. Thus, the lobbyists for these industries have created a defensive shell of disinformation to protect their interests. Governments and public health bodies may not even really want to win the war against excess weight; there are too many private interests at stake. That's why we hear double-talk from decision-makers who condemn the epidemic but offer no solutions, or worse, who propose poor solutions that are doomed to fail.

Consumer culture, the cause of weight problems, undermines all of our attempts to remedy them, no matter how much suffering they cause. Do we have to throw up our hands in defeat? No. I developed the plan contained in this book to address these enormous obstacles with a new and different approach: by preventing excess weight from developing in the first place.

Throughout this book, I address the reader directly. The power to stop the deadly epidemic is in your hands. During pregnancy, the siren call of consumption will be drowned out by the instinct to care for the child in your womb. With the help of the plan I will outline for you in Chapter 5, I believe you'll be fully prepared to actively protect your unborn child during its primary development and prevent it from forming a lifelong susceptibility.

But now, let's return to the dangers of being overweight, its consequences, and its complications. The aim is not to scare you, but simply to describe the enemy from every angle. And it's important to remember one thing: weight problems are as dangerous as they are avoidable.

Complications Resulting from Excess Weight and Obesity

The consequences are many: They are linked with a vast range of pathologies. Quite simply, an obese person is 10 times more at risk of having a weight-related disease than a non-obese person.

Type 2 Diabetes

This section will be of particular interest if there are diabetics in your family, you're seriously overweight, you have previously suffered from gestational diabetes, or you eat a lot of sugary foods or fast carbohydrates like white bread, white rice, white pasta, or potatoes.

Diabetes is by far the most direct complication of being overweight. This has led to its being grouped under a broad new category: diabesity. The concept was created because obesity and diabetes have the same origin: both are caused by insulin and the pancreas that secretes it. The vast majority of type 2 diabetics are overweight or obese.

The danger of diabetes lies in the fact that it's a silent condition that emerges once the damage, which often comes in multiple forms, already poses a serious threat.

Diabetes emerges when the pancreas loses control of glucose concentration in the blood. At a blood glucose level of around 100 mg/dl, glucose is necessary and, in fact, indispensable. But beyond a blood glucose level of 115 mg/dl, it becomes increasingly corrosive for many organs. At a fasting blood glucose level of 126 mg/dl, diabetes is already present.

If it weren't for the pancreas, however—if we didn't have insulin—glucose would be deadly, at a blood glucose level of about 700 to 1,000 mg/dl. A diabetic whose pancreas has shut down and who is taking insulin and forgets to take their treatment would go into a diabetic coma and die in less than an hour after consuming half a loaf of French bread and a soda.

Complications of Diabetes

Heart attack. Heart attacks strike diabetics three to four times more often than nondiabetics. A diabetic heart attack is often silent, since nerve damage reduces the sensation of pain, which means that diagnosis and treatment tend to be delayed. In the acute phase of a heart attack, insulin is injected to lower the amount of blood sugar attacking the heart. The gravity of having too much glucose is all too clear.

Blindness. Diabetes is the leading cause of acquired blindness. A prolonged excess of glucose in the blood damages the small capillaries and arterioles that deliver nutrients to the retina. This causes edema, dilation, and bleeding, which eventually lead to blindness.

Once again, glucose is the culprit. And, as always, high glucose levels are caused by failure of the pancreas and its resulting inability to secrete insulin.

Arterial hypertension. This condition is so commonly associated with diabetes that it's almost considered an inherent symptom. Arterial hypertension affects one out of two diabetics. This condition, in combination with excess weight localized on the paunch and diabetes, sets the stage for metabolic syndrome, a cluster of health risks that occur together, such as high blood sugar, high blood pressure, and high triglyceride level, increasing the risk for heart disease, stroke, and diabetes.

Hypertension worsens the prognosis of diabetes by accelerating the onset of heart attack and, especially, stroke.

Kidney damage. Sugar is the most common and most damaging toxin for the kidneys, and diabetes is the number one cause of kidney failure. Those who suffer from kidney failure must use a dialysis machine to rid the body of its waste.

We often hear that proteins damage the kidneys. This unfounded rumor is just a diversion used by the sugar industry. It's meant to distract us from the fact that the only nutrient that alters the kidney is sugar. Kidney damage occurs when blood glucose levels exceed 140 mg/dl.

Vulnerability in the womb. If you're pregnant, you probably already know that an adult's nutritional needs differ from a child's, and even more so from those of a newborn. But the difference is greater still when it comes to a fetus undergoing intensive development.

During the months of your pregnancy, you have to pay close attention to the information you take in, particularly when it comes to advertising messages. The gatekeepers for advertising rate the truth and risks of messages about food products according to their consumption by *adults,* not considering their *effect on an unborn child* carried by an adult woman.

While it takes decades for sugars to profoundly affect an adult's health, this is not the case for a growing fetus. As the fetus incorporates the diet of the woman who carries it, its developing pancreas is at risk of being disrupted at a crucial moment. This will cause a vulnerability that will make the risks from sugars greater and potentially more harmful.

Nerve damage. Nerve damage from sugar is one of the most common complications from diabetes. It occurs when prolonged excess of glucose attacks the nerves and profoundly impairs their functioning. One of the worst and most common problems is its effect on sensitivity to pain. Intense pain can be caused merely by contact between a piece of cloth and the foot; or, numbness can occur, making sufferers unaware that they're being burned or injured. This explains why many infected wounds suffered by diabetics end up requiring amputation. Reduced sugar consumption and glycemic control (control of blood sugar) can diminish this complication if the onset of diabetes is recent. If it's not, controlling sugar can only stabilize the condition.

Diabetes and amputation. When diabetes is managed poorly over a long period of time, atherosclerosis may occur. The condition results in less oxygen-rich arterial blood reaching the extremities. Just a tiny wound, recognized too late due to a loss of sensitivity, can lead to infections that don't heal. Atherosclerosis is a breeding ground for small gangrenes of the big toe, the foot, and to some extent, the leg. Seventy percent of non-accidental amputations are caused by diabetes.

Diabetes and male erection. Diabetes is the leading organic cause of erectile dysfunction. According to *Diabetes Québec*, 50 to 75 percent of diabetic men lose their ability to maintain erection, and suffer from sexual problems.

A normal erection is caused by blood being trapped in the cavernous tissue of the penis. For a sufficient and sustainable erection, it is essential that the arteries, veins, nerves, and male hormones play their role perfectly.

With diabetics, however, high glucose levels damage the arterial, venous, and nervous systems. Furthermore, being overweight encourages the conversion of the male hormone testosterone into the female hormone estrogen. When complications from diabetes arise, the mounting problems often lead to a state of depression, which, combined with erectile dysfunction, can cause relationship problems for couples.

Sleep apnea. Sleep apnea consists of pauses in breathing during deep sleep. Breathing stops for more than 10 seconds, more than five times an hour. These apneas have a profound effect on quality of life, causing debilitating fatigue, headaches, and drowsiness while awake.

In obese patients, weight gain affects the base of the tongue, which is very rich in adipose tissue. The increased weight of the tongue puts pressure on the larynx, reducing its diameter to the point of obstruction. Sleep apnea sufferers often experience slackening and loss of muscle tone in the throat and larynx, which aggravates the obstruction.

Joint pain. Excess weight puts mechanical stress on cartilage, wearing it out faster. The most sensitive joints and those most often affected are the knees, as well as the lumbar vertebrae, and, for those who are predisposed, the hips. Before resorting to drug therapy or surgery, rheumatologists and orthopedic surgeons ask their patients to lose weight. Patients tend to comply, since losing weight quickly improves symptoms.

When diabetes is a factor, other symptoms appear that tend to be misdiagnosed. The increase in glucose damages and weakens the tendons. In combination with their excess weight, diabetics suffer from multiple tendinitis problems that disrupt their motor skills and cause night pain that affects quality of sleep.

Alzheimer's. Diabetics are one and a half to two times more likely to develop Alzheimer's. Toxicity from excess sugar in the blood also affects the brain. The extra glucose attacks micro-circulation and alters the neurons. Furthermore, resistance to insulin leads to inflammatory stress, which adds to the effects on nerve cells. Finally, the body neutralizes the excess glucose by transforming it into triglycerides, which contribute to neurons being damaged by amyloid plaques.

Alzheimer's specialists today believe that a diet low in sugar, along with physical activity that consumes glucose, delays the onset of the disease.

Risks to Heart

The heart is especially vulnerable to excess weight.

First, in people suffering from obesity, the exertion required for the heart to pump is directly correlated to the amount of excess weight a person has. Carrying just a 20-pound backpack can raise the heart rate and increase the strength of cardiac contraction in an individual who is unfit.

Second, excess fat creates a resistance to blood flow. More fat means the heart muscle has to pump harder to get through areas where fat is concentrated. This creates an increase in blood pressure.

In the arteries, obesity and diabetes are very often related to high triglycerides and "bad" blood cholesterol, as well as lower "good" cholesterol. The combined effect of the problems is clogging of the arteries and weakening of their walls.

The combination of narrowed arteries weakened by atherosclerotic plaques and blood circulating under high pressure creates the conditions for dangerous circulatory events in areas where vascularization is essential. One example would be in the coronary arteries, which deliver nutrients to the heart; the closing of these arteries causes angina and heart attack.

Stroke

In obese individuals and diabetics, the large carotid arteries that reach up the neck to carry blood to the brain often become partially obstructed. The same goes for the entire cerebral arterial system. Under these strenuous conditions, all it takes is poorly managed or ignored hypertension (high blood pressure) for an artery to become blocked, or worse, ruptured, to cause bleeding and compression of the brain.

Cancer

Today, we have total scientific consensus on the direct links between cancer and diet. According to the European CanCer Organisation (ECCO), a European anticancer organization, almost half a million new cases of cancer among adults worldwide can be attributed to excess weight and obesity. Among the known factors, one of the most of common is excess weight and diabetes.

We know that sugar and invasive carbohydrates end up in the blood in the form of glucose, and we know that glucose plays a key role in the development and propagation of cancer. But how does this occur?

Let's compare a normal cell and a cancerous cell. A normal cell functions in a hybrid mode: its nutrients are glucose and fatty acids (from sugar or fat). A cancerous cell, however, doesn't use fat. *Its sole nutrient is glucose, which it needs to survive.*

However, glucose does more than just fuel the multiplication and dissemination of cancerous cells. It also causes the reflexive production of insulin, which indirectly triggers the production of insulin-like growth factor (IGF), a powerful protein that stimulates the growth of cancerous cells. Finally (as if all that wasn't enough), we know that hypertrophic fat cells in overweight or obese individuals experience stress and produce cytokines, which create inflammation.

For all these reasons, most oncologists today recommend to their patients a diet low in invasive sugars, which slows down tumor development and, especially, metastasis, the spread of cancer.

Depression

Obesity and diabetes are now recognized as twin conditions; they fall under the new concept of diabesity. Combined, the two conditions commonly lead to dissatisfaction, suffering, and anxiety. These, in turn, are statistically linked to a third condition, one that is also spreading rapidly: depression.

The Prevalence of Comorbid Depression in Adults with Diabetes, a large study published in *Diabetic Medicine* in 2006, showed that diabetics are twice as likely to suffer from depression than non-diabetics are. The association has more to do with the psychological impact of the disease than with its metabolic factors. The proof: undiagnosed diabetics or those unaware of their condition are less likely to be depressed than those who are aware.

As for excess weight, a large study by Leiden University found that obesity promotes depression, and depression in turn leads to weight gain. Specifically, obese individuals have an almost 55 percent risk of developing depression, and people suffering from depression have a 58 percent risk of becoming obese.

The accumulation of excess weight, especially when it reaches the obesity stage, can create a feeling of exclusion and lack of self-worth. The sense of rejecting one's body and self-image, and the feeling (real or imagined) of being discriminated against, can lead to complexes, inhibition, and loss of self-esteem.

Then, there's the flip side of the coin. People with depression tend to feel a desperate need for satisfaction. They tend to find this satisfaction in sugary and fatty foods, which cause weight gain.

Depression also diminishes a person's motivation to stick to a diet program or diabetes management regimen, just as it impairs compliance with medication and, especially, physical activity.

Finally, to make matters worse, most antidepressants cause weight gain.

Maternal Instinct

In this chapter, I have tried to present the enemy—excess weight, obesity, and diabetes—in its true colors. The enemy has a special power: Those who suffer from it or are threatened believe, with good reason, that they can evade the threat at any moment. They can therefore wait for another day to make a change. But delaying can lead to dire results.

I created the plan laid out in this book because I am convinced that the unbelievable explosion in excess weight around the world is in large part due to the rise in the number of children who are affected by a vulnerability to weight problems and diabetes that they acquired in their mother's womb. This vulnerability remains when these children grow up and become adults. A diet too high in refined sugars has generated a new model of human being: one that is infinitely more prone to gaining weight and becoming diabetic. It's this process that helps explain how the population of overweight people has risen from several hundred million to over two billion. In 1980, there were 100 million diabetics in the world; today, the number has soared to more than 400 million.

But there's reason for optimism. If you are pregnant, you are the sole link between the food you eat and the glucose that ends up in the blood and pancreas of your child. Therefore, you are naturally the only person who can ensure your child's dietary protection. And you can ensure this protection if you understand why and how to avoid glucose-related problems. My mission is to help you become aware of that necessity and give you the right tools to succeed.

The food production industry and its powerful army of advertisers don't set out to willfully harm anyone. But they are driven by a single objective: to produce profit as efficiently as possible. During the crucial months of pregnancy, this plan will show you how to distinguish foods that are tolerable for you but not for your child. It isn't easy to maintain a critical stance while watching highly seductive television commercials. You need to stay on guard.

It's common for a commercial to convince you that you really want a sugary cookie loaded with flour. You may think you need that snack to stay alert and compensate for the energy you've lost over the morning. But your maternal instinct can alert you it's a trap and keep you from falling into that trap. To take just one example, one of the best-selling cookies in France is 62 percent carbohydrates and almost 20 percent white sugar. And yet, incredibly, this cookie is presented as weight-loss friendly.

Before writing this book, I spent a lot of time reflecting. I was reluctant to join in this struggle; I've had sufficient experience with lobbies to know how powerful they are, and to know that this plan would be much more of a target for attack than my diet was. That's because this plan attacks the problem at the root. It therefore poses a serious threat to the activities and the profits of a very powerful industry.

My hope is that the more the epidemic spreads and the more costly and alienating it becomes, the more consumers will rise up to form a resistance against the suffering it causes. The day will come when the producers learn that their economic model has sprung a leak and that their own survival depends on shifting the paradigm. The process is already underway. In 2014, annual sales for The Coca-Cola Company and McDonald's actually declined. (Coca-Cola dropped 1.37 percent to reach $12.57 billion: a far cry from the $12.87 billion expected. McDonald's had a similar result, with sales of $7.18 billion, lower than the $7.29 anticipated.)

But this evolution may take time. In the argument I propose in this book, I have an ally—a very powerful ally. It's the maternal instinct. I've witnessed enough women quit smoking or drinking without hesitation upon learning that they are pregnant. I'm convinced that if I can pass on my beliefs and the results of my research, all the lobbies combined couldn't hide the truth.

Chapter 2

The Causes of Excess Weight, Obesity, and Diabetes

Every mother-to-be should know the reasons for excess weight, obesity, and diabetes to protect her child. You're probably seeing that as we explore the different complications caused by excess weight, the same culprit keeps popping up: excess sugar.

A category of foods appeared quite recently. Foods rich in proteins (meats, fish, etc.) and foods rich in fats (oils and butter) haven't changed much. Carbohydrates, particularly those that have been modified and processed by the food industry, have become ubiquitous. The existence of essential amino acids and fatty acids proves that proteins and fats are vital nutrients—we need them to live. Conversely, the lack of the equivalent acids for carbohydrates tells us that there *is no such thing as essential carbohydrates*. Each step of industrial processing makes carbohydrates more penetrating and invasive. When they flood the bloodstream, they abruptly raise blood glucose levels, requiring the pancreas to secrete ever more insulin. Insulin, in turn, leads to weight gain by transforming glucose into fat. The pancreas, being overworked, can eventually become exhausted, which opens the door to diabetes.

Only a very strong pancreas can deal with such aggressive and artificial foods. This strength is developed during the last six months of pregnancy. To achieve it, it is essential that the fetus's tiny pancreas, which develops so rapidly, be given the chance to grow without being bombarded by an excessive amount of these foods. This is why maternal nutrition plays such a determining role on the pancreas of an unborn child.

Here are three little-known reasons for the current weight crisis:

1. Excess weight and obesity aren't a focus in the medical field; they are not confronted and taken seriously by physicians until they reach the complication stage. So long as excess weight does not immediately threaten life or health, it is seen as a trivial matter, a subject for magazines and fitness gurus. Unfortunately, however, when the complications arise, they are serious and difficult to reverse.

2. Excess weight is a result of the intersection of supply and demand. On one side is the compulsive craving for foods that provide quick gratification. On the other side is an abundant supply of an ever-expanding selection of appealing products. People who become overweight suffer as their bodies change, but the suffering seems minor compared with the suffering they would experience if they deprived themselves of the weight-causing products.

3. The invasion of industrially produced, highly processed carbohydrates is encountered by a pancreas that came into being in a

time before it could be designed or evolve in such a way to deal with them.

When the glucose in your blood rises from 100 mg/dl to just 200 mg/dl, the blood becomes seriously toxic to all the organs it irrigates. As a response, this blood sugar is transformed into fat, which leads to excess weight and, eventually, diabetes.

Producers that control food supplies have only one objective: to convince consumers to buy their products. They have two ways of achieving this. The first employs the classic logic of seduction and competition through marketing, packaging, and advertising. The second is infinitely more insidious. It focuses on undermining the natural foundations for human happiness, which I'll discuss in more detail later in this chapter. This is because *unhappy consumers consume more than happy consumers.*

But this same market logic also offers hope. Industry profits depend on us playing our role as consumers. If we choose to purchase healthy food products, the industry will respond. It will provide more of the products we want.

The Weight Crisis: A Recent Struggle between the Individual and Society

We are about to enter a subject area that should be of interest to everyone, especially mothers-to-be. Strap on your seat belt. We will look at two inseparable and complementary sides of our human world: the individual and society. Each has its own program to follow. But it is the recent opposition between the two that is at the origin of weight problems and decreased happiness.

The Primary Role of the Individual

At a very early stage of your life, during the first months in utero, an initial command was issued within the hypothalamus—one of the deepest and most archaic parts of the brain, a part we share with reptiles. If life were compared to an ultra-sophisticated computer program, this command would be the first and fundamental rule of the program: live.

Let's say that command was given to a transmitter that we will call the life pulsar. The life pulsar could be compared to an embryo's heart, which starts to beat at around the same period. The pulsar transmits the simple need or appetite for life. It's what makes you get up every morning without questioning the instinct to enjoy the world and build a life for yourself. As with hunger or thirst or sexual desire, the will to live is driven by energy, desire, and motivation, and it moves you more powerfully when you're preparing to bring new life into the world.

This motivating energy naturally flows into different channels, resulting in a number of behaviors being expressed. These behaviors are very familiar to each of us: their job is to keep us alive. Neurologists call them reward-seeking behaviors.

I believe that this reward system is probably one of the keys to the evolution of life, and the system probably became part of the evolution of our species at its very origins. Incredibly simple and amazingly effective, it has persisted over countless generations and is still very present today. *The more useful a behavior is for the protection and perpetuation of life, the more reward it earns; the more reward it earns, the more the behavior is desirable and practiced.*

But it goes even further. Behaviors that are favorable to a given species are selected and integrated into its very DNA. The first of these behaviors is centered on the need to feed oneself. This need is a condition for existence; without it, everything quickly grinds to a halt. The benefit is big, and hence, the reward is, too.

But the intensity of this need varies from person to person. On rare occasions, I've encountered patients who, while not anorexic, don't experience the drive to eat. These individuals take in nourishment only in order to survive.

The same thing happens with sexual desire—a need associated with love, the pleasure of giving life and protecting it, and which provides a major reward. A widespread repulsion toward sex would spell the end of our species.

Reward and the circuits through which it is provided are not limited to these two needs. During my professional life, I've met with patients who are unable to switch off their exacerbated need to eat; in monitoring these patients, I discovered that they had difficulty satisfying other human needs, and that they compensated for their dissatisfaction by eating more food as a reward.

I followed this line of investigation further. My work was guided by considering the lives of early man and the last Neanderthals, and even the great apes. My goal was essentially to identify and understand our reasons for living.

In this way, I was gradually able to identify 10 fundamental needs (page 35) that are inscribed in the human genetic code, or DNA.

Satisfying the 10 fundamental needs gives us rewards; it provides a beneficial and fulfilling experience while ensuring life and survival.

Our genes, the start of our childhood, the culture that surrounds us, our place and our moment in history, and encounters we have with others all result in some of our reward channels opening up and others narrowing or completely closing off. It is not necessary to use all our reward channels in order to live; we can function with just three or four.

When a reward-seeking behavior is successful, the reward appears. This is manifested at two levels simultaneously:

- The first is the sense of enjoying life, of experiencing good feelings, from simple contentment to pleasure to euphoria and the unfurling of energy that results, the kind that makes you leap for joy and cry out with happiness.

- The second is strictly biological and functions unconsciously. The reward is expressed by an intracerebral secretion of two chemical mediators: dopamine and serotonin. The primary function of

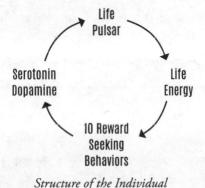

Structure of the Individual

these two substances is to return to the life pulsar—to recharge it, so to speak. The energy that was emitted thus ends up back at the beginning of the circuit. These two chemical mediators are commonly cited to explain dependence and addiction.

So, in summary: the life pulsar emits energy that activates the reward circuits. This releases dopamine and serotonin, which close the circuit by making their return to the pulsar for recharging.

It's this circuit that keeps human life going.

The Primary Role of Society

Human society consists of a group of individuals living and working together. It could be compared to a human body; like cells, individuals cooperate to form the social body.

During the very long period when humankind lived as hunter-gatherers, human societies were made up of 50 to 200 people. With the emergence of civilization, societies became progressively larger, eventually expanding to include millions of people.

A society obviously doesn't have the same physical embodiment as an individual, but it is governed by analogous rules. Like the individual, society is driven by its own pulsar. However, the social pulsar is not a fixed part of our genetic framework. It can be altered.

That's what happened in 1944 when a cultural revolution introduced a radically new pulsar. This change resulted in a new model of civilization, one that deeply uprooted society and the lives and development of its members.

In that year, at the end of the war, the shaken allied countries gathered, at the invitation of the United States, in Bretton Woods, a small town in New Hampshire, at the United Nations Monetary and Financial Conference. The objective was to rebuild their economies.

It was in this context of rebuilding that the concept of indefinite growth was born. The trials of the war and feats of technology instilled a powerful hope for prosperity and happiness. The concept of permanent growth was born from this hope. This concept became the foundation of our societies—it was the social equivalent of the life pulsar for the individual.

The primary command of the individual life pulsar is *live*; that of society is *grow indefinitely, and more each year*. A growing society is one that creates more wealth, goods, and services than it did the previous year. But to produce more upstream, it is necessary that there are consumers downstream who will absorb the surplus produced.

This totally new model became known as the consumer society.

So long as it was a matter of meeting basic human needs, the opportunity for this consumption was considered a blessing. Human society welcomed elevators, vehicles, new medications and means of communication. Intense physical effort was gradually eradicated.

Once the more basic needs were covered, other comfort-providing products appeared: appliances, washing machines, dishwashers, and many more, all of which were equally welcomed.

Eventually, consumers started to feel that their needs were met. They were ready to take a relaxed breath from consuming. But this threatened to disrupt the system.

To maintain the rate of consumption—household demand, as it is famously known—society flew to the rescue of the great production machine. The solution was to develop two types of incentives that would push consumer temptation to new levels.

One, a positive incentive: the classical component of selling a product, based on cosmetic seduction. Marketing, packaging, advertising, "As Seen on TV"; all these come together and form a collective attack to promote impulse buys.

Two, a negative incentive: a deeply immoral one, which aims to do nothing less than distance individuals from the satisfaction of the 10 fundamental needs, those that are most natural and human, in order to push them toward instead consumption.

Why?

Of those 10 fundamental needs, eight are free. Consider the powerful need covered by the term "sexuality," most broadly speaking, which includes love and family. Loving one's wife, mother, or children is basic, natural, and powerful, and it does not involve consumption. The consumption industry aligns itself with anything that can break the hold of these fundamental needs.

Two of these 10 needs can be profitable: the need for food and the need for play. Food products sell extremely well, since they provide a sensory experience and have been made addictive with the inclusion of processed ingredients. Play and recreation provide the joy of having fun, laughing, dancing, and singing with other humans. This need for play has been diverted from its primary function to become an object of consumption. Today, it is becoming solitary and passive, delivered by TV screens, electronic games, and entertainment on demand. It sells extremely well.

For the past 50 years, the engagement between our hearts and the world around us is quietly and progressively eroding. We are beginning to feel comfortable forgetting the smell of trees, eradicating physical effort, relegating beauty to walled-in museums, encasing spirituality in steel and concrete, restricting the pleasure of rewarding work to a lucky elite, and turning from group belonging to consumer individualism, whose pleasures are wrapped in a plastic package.

The shift results from a structural change to our place in the world. With the vastness and complexity of an overpopulated planet in which life expectancy has doubled, a new society has emerged. This society has come to dominate the individual in order to achieve maximum sales growth.

This new society depends on the economy and technology for its survival. As the great social machine turns, its fundamental strategy is transmitted to each of its "gears":

The first gear is the consumption industry. This industry, in turn, determines the movements of the second gear, the decision-makers: politicians, economists, financiers, advertisers, media, unions, and even the unemployed, who receive support.

Inevitably, this great machine turns at the expense of human beings. It creates a way of life that seems extraordinarily rich and stimulating but is artificial and cold. It replaces full and profound natural satisfactions with artificial ones that are superficial and ephemeral. Consumers must be constantly surprised, ever more frequently and intensely, in order to remain interested. As our civilization speeds ever forward, constant innovation is necessary to maintain the stimulating thrill of tearing into a new package.

As time goes on, the products that once provided satisfaction no longer produce the same feeling of reward. Consumers in the social group begin to prefer immediate satisfaction, and once familiar purchases fail to produce the same rewards. The satisfactions based on consumption are therefore unable to produce dopamine and serotonin, the chemicals that fuel the love of life.

When low levels of serotonin persist or worsen, so does the lust for life, and the risk of falling below the minimum limits of satisfaction arises. This is the realm of unhappiness and depression.

The satisfaction of these needs is instantaneous and easily available: We get it from eating food and looking at screens. Too much food rich in invasive carbohydrates and too much time spent motionless in front of screens leads to weight gain, which propels the weight crisis forward. This shift is hard to control when the consumer society goes along with it. The individual and society could continue to function together in this way, with great efficiency. But at a certain point, a fundamental break between them is possible—and it's crucial to remember this point as we move forward.

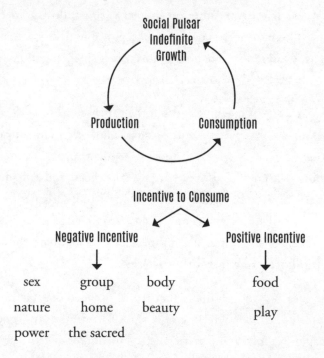

Structure of Society

Ancient Mind vs. New Mind

Each of us essentially has two minds: an ancient mind and a new mind. The new mind produces and manages consciousness, culture, technology, and progress. Indeed, this is the mind that first envisioned and designed the new world of consumption. The ancient mind manages the functioning of the body, emotions, pleasure, and above all, *survival.* Our survival absolutely depends on the love of life, instilled through the secretion of serotonin and dopamine, which is regulated by the reward circuit.

10 Fundamental Needs

I developed this theory over the course of my professional life. Most of my patients who come to me because they want to lose weight tell me about the suffering they endure because of that weight. But they continue to eat in a way that can only prolong the problem.

Without their realizing it, these men and women clearly eat as they do to alleviate the suffering they experience unconsciously.

Observing animals has shown us that when animals face stress, suffering, or a threat, they try to make it stop or they flee to escape it. When fight-or-flight isn't an option, they opt for a third solution: they try to obtain pleasure in order to neutralize the displeasure.

Psychologists have tried to explain weight problems by looking at individual vulnerability related to childhood and early trauma. This argument is perfectly valid when it comes to explaining any given person's history. But not all of the 26 million overweight people in France—almost seven million of whom are obese—can blame a difficult childhood. A social cause has to be at the heart of this epidemic.

Most of my patients who are affected by excess weight are suffering, not always in a conscious or perceived way, but due to vulnerability and hypersensitivity to stress and life's challenges.

To understand the origin of this suffering, I focused on their personal histories. What I discovered was significant events or failures, often with multiple origins. Most often they included emotional difficulties, family problems, and ruptured relationships. I often encountered professional problems as well, such as the inability to flourish in the workplace. Then there was a sedentary lifestyle, loss of connection with their body, isolation, spiritual emptiness, lack of self-confidence, and low self-esteem, all colored by a mood of depression.

With time and by gaining the trust of my patients, I was able to trace back the multiple origins of this suffering. In doing so, I was able to identify, one by one, those 10 fundamental needs that, when unsatisfied, cause people to seek a substitute feeling of satisfaction through food.

1. Sexuality in the broadest sense, including love and family.

Sexuality, love, and family constitute a major need. Problems within couples, divorces, estrangements from children, loneliness, and lack of sexual relationships can generate profound suffering. Many patients who see me for weight problems or obesity have told me that their weight gain took place in a context of emotional difficulties, and that losing weight and keeping it off was much easier than dealing with these issues.

2. Satisfaction in work.

Time and again, my patients gained a lot of weight following problems in their professional lives and difficulty succeeding in their work. Some had lost their jobs and were experiencing humiliation from being unemployed. I also met with patients who had been left disoriented by retirement and struggled with a sensation of uselessness and boredom. Most often, however, the men and women I spoke with found their work to lack joy, responsibility, room for creativity, or connection with other humans. Work was simply a way to put food on the table—one that required too much travel time.

The need to succeed in work and to reach professional heights can be so intense that it ends up obstructing other sources of satisfaction. But happiness is too meaningful and too important to be fully accessible via a single door. I've met with prominent captains of industry, people of great wealth and power, who are missing that one essential component of life.

Just as life's ups and downs have an impact on sexuality, an improvement in an individual's professional life can lead to a reduction in compulsive eating.

3. Safety and comfort of home.

In speaking to patients, I discovered the impact of home on maintaining a sense of balance and fulfillment. I noticed the importance of a safe and comfortable place where we can feel at home—a space to decorate the way we want, come together with people we care about, and feel peace and calm.

Housing-related problems are anything but trivial. A long distance from work, a lack of safety, the stress of city life, the ugliness of buildings, an estrangement from nature, and the exorbitant costs per square foot; all have an impact on quality of life.

When the most comfortable area of the home centers around the refrigerator, the kitchen cupboards, and the TV screen, it creates a cocktail that has powerful repercussions on weight.

4. The need for play.

One constant in my life has been a keen interest in primitive man and ethology, the study of animal behavior. Throughout my career, I've explored the origin of humankind, examining everything from philosophy to medicine. As a young student, I worked with the zoologist and future Nobel Prize winner Konrad Lorenz. I was fascinated with this legendary man, who was famous for his unique skill as a "goose whisperer." Reading his work taught me that the vast majority of social animals are equipped with a need to play.

Lorenz saw in animal play the foundation for group bonds; he also believed play was a source of joy and a way to facilitate the ability to learn. It's clear to anyone who watches young lion clubs at play that the young animals are actually forming relationships. It's also clear that their tentative use of claws and fangs are a way to acquire, at a very young age, the gestures and postures they will use in combat. They are learning to kill. The need for play seemed so universal that it must have a crucial function.

In tandem with my medical studies, I was very inspired by anthropology courses taught by André Leory-Gouran and ethnology courses taught by Claude Lévi-Strauss. Their work confirmed that the animal need to play reached its culmination in humankind.

Among the Inuit, nights are spent in igloos, with everyone gathered around the fire for hours on end. The time is spent playing, miming, teasing, and telling jokes, as one clan member states: "We tell the same stories to make everyone laugh every night: the story of a cousin who slipped on the ice, or who let the best seal of the year get away."

This need to play is another aspect of life that seems to be languishing. We all know that we are compelled by play. But the consumerist model tirelessly trivializes any activity that is simple and doesn't have a price tag, such as children's games of hopscotch or old-fashioned dance parties, as having no apparent use.

Our great desire for play has largely been overtaken by the passive and solitary spectacle of screens that display television shows and electronic games. The lack of play that involves interaction with other people leads to frustration. This may be less obvious than the frustration related to sex or food.

Play, laughter, and joy distract us. They create intervals suspended from other parts of our life. These intervals offer the chance to let anxiety and daily stresses fade. For the seventeenth-century philosopher Pascal, recreation is one of the best strategies evolution has given us to allow us to forget—at least for a while—that life comes to an end: "A king without diversion is a man sunk into wretchedness." As I've often found, a similar fact is true for my patients: boredom causes hunger.

5. Belonging to a group.

Once again, it was primitive man and the great apes that pointed me toward this need, which has been drowned in today's mega-societies.

Remember that for a need to enter into a species' genetic code, it must have shown that it aids the survival of the species and its members. Such is the case with the need to belong to a group, a need that all social animals display. Interestingly, each group has a critical mass according to species. The optimal number depends on various characteristics, such as anatomy, living territory, or nutritional needs. A pack of bloodthirsty wolves is better equipped when hunting as a large group; a group of gorillas whose only aim is to eat tasty bamboo can be small in number. But whatever their size and number, all social animals feel the need to belong to a group.

Jane Goodall, who spent a great deal of time among chimpanzees, found that for these animals, belonging to a group is absolutely vital. Any chimpanzee rejected from its group is doomed to die. Death can occur physically, at the teeth of a predator, but also emotionally, from the trauma of being excluded from its group—like a cell or an organ separated from a body.

Of all these animals, however, humans have the strongest need for a group. Humans lack claws and fangs that provide defense or the ability to hunt. Ever since we left the trees and abandoned a fruit-based diet, we have survived, for millions of years, through cooperation within a group.

But this need for a collective is undermined by urban life and the gigantic size of today's societies, which are dictated by a culture of individualism. Cultivating our intelligence, or accumulating and disseminating knowledge, can make our animal need for human groups seem obsolete. We may also feel that we no longer need groups to feed ourselves, defend ourselves, or experience play. Yet, we still need to obtain the satisfaction (limited as it may be) that comes from being part of a group. If we don't get that satisfaction, we deprive ourselves of a reward that the brain must then seek elsewhere. Failing to satisfy this need means we deprive ourselves the pleasure of connection and familiarity and the extra serotonin and dopamine that result, nourishing the desire to live.

Fortunately, there are those who find fulfillment and self-expression in the group. These people take joy in connecting with and helping others. They usually focus first and foremost on their circle of friends and family. When they find this inner circle to be a reliable source of connection, they include others.

Many of my patients, however, experience this sense of belonging only in a limited way through the choices and slogans that create a bond among an anonymous group of consumers. Some manage to avoid alienation by affirming their humanity within humanitarian, charitable, environmental, or political associations that offer a path to fulfillment. But others who fail to find such means are deprived of a powerful source of satisfaction. They may unconsciously turn to other sources of natural satisfaction, the most simple and powerful of which is food.

6 Using the body.

This is the need that is the most obvious of all, but surprisingly, is the least understood and attended to. I discovered this powerful need by reading *Spark,* a book by American psychiatrist John J. Ratey, who undertook a thorough study of the relationship between physical and mental activity.

Ratey is one of a number of researchers who have shown the public and the medical community the extent of the organic links between physical activity and depression, stress management, hyperactivity, and anxiety disorders.

It's an oft-repeated fact that physical activity is good for your health. In fact, it's more than good for you. It's indispensable, and not just for the reasons that are usually mentioned.

To understand the essence of the need for physical activity and the reasons for that need, you have to look deeper. Animals are different from plants since they have neither roots nor leaves, and must move around to find food and reproduce. For this activity to be effective, animals need a brain to direct and guide them.

Neuroscientists who have worked in this field have discovered, and recently proven, that physical activity in humans and animals leads to the release of serotonin. This is shown by studies conducted with groups of patients suffering from severe depression. These studies compared the effects of Zoloft, a popular antidepressant, with the effects of physical activity. The results showed that the two treatments were comparable in terms of efficacy.

Nowadays this is a well-known fact for most doctors, but the majority of people are still convinced that physical activity is only good for burning calories and fighting obesity.

But what's much less known and fascinating to neuroscientists today is that physical activity releases not just serotonin but also brain-derived neurotrophic factor (BDNF). BDNF is a growth factor that protects neurons by slowing their decline; it therefore protects memory.

And there's a lot more. One of the most firmly rooted dogmas of twentieth-century neurology is that we come into the world with a limited number of neurons, and that starting from the end of early childhood, we lose them each day, with no hope of getting more. In 1998, however, this dogma was shattered by the chance discovery that certain parts of the brain could create new nerve cells from stem cells.

This neuronal regeneration is controlled by BDNF, and physical activity stimulates its release. This represents a great hope for the possibility of delaying or mitigating degenerative brain diseases, such as Alzheimer's or Parkinson's.

At another level, seemingly far removed from the topic of serious diseases, consider that only 30 minutes of jogging or 1 hour of walking per day improves not only your mood but also your intellectual power.

For all these reasons, engaging your body is one of the fundamental needs whose satisfaction offers a wealth of fulfillment. It's part of the formula for happiness. Yet the majority of patients who come to see me for obesity, excess weight, or diabetes are extremely sedentary. A sedentary lifestyle is an inherent part of our way of life today, when one out of two patents filed is intended to save time or reduce physical activity. This widespread dependence on effort-saving technology increasingly makes physical activity a thing of the past, relegating it to the status of a task or chore. Certainly, it may be possible to survive with an extremely low level of activity. But doing so deprives us of a proven, undeniable source of satisfaction.

7. Experiencing nature.

Humans need nature; we ourselves are an element of nature. There's no need to wax philosophical or moral to explain it. Brain imaging has shown that immersion in nature, whether it's walking in the forest or near the ocean, near plants and animals, activates the reward centers of the brain. Yet we've come to think that urban life has more value and utility, that nature just doesn't provide the same visual and auditory stimulation.[1]

In 2012, the Organisation for Economic Co-operation and Development (OECD) estimated that 70 percent of the world's population would be living in urban areas by 2050.

And yet, once again, there's a vast difference between what culture tells us and what nature shows us. Trees, flowers, leaves, forests, the sky and clouds, wind and storms, the ocean with its waves and their salty spray, the soil, sand, rivers, and wild animals fascinate us because we are programmed to hear, see, and smell them. Each moment

---

1   In 1960, 33.6 percent of the world's population lived in urban areas; in 2014, the percentage was 53.4. Source: World Bank (http://databank.banquemondiale.org/data/home.aspx).

nature calls to us and every message it emits to us is recognized by our ancient mind, our instinctual side, as a sign that we belong and are connected to *life*.

So how do we connect with nature today? René Char, a renowned French poet and philosopher, wrote to me one day with an observation: "Forests are sleeping within our gardens." For most of us, gardens have become a luxury. But something as simple as a potted geranium on a balcony is a link.

Pets are another outlet for our need for nature. And there are others: an overcrowded beach that's nonetheless a sanctuary for nature, a children's park or garden, or spots for hunting or fishing.

But all these things share a single disadvantage: they are free. That means there's no incentive for businesses to encourage us to enjoy our happiness. Experiencing nature is a simple way to create satisfaction and the desire to live.

But there's reason to have hope. This need can easily be reappropriated, brought back to the forefront of our lives; it can even be boosted by combining it with physical activity. It's easy to run or walk in a forest or barefoot on the sand, or to bring a domesticated animal into your life, from a horse you can ride to a dog that can protect your home to a cat that can offer warmth and affection.

8. Spirituality and transcendence.

You may have noticed that all the needs we've looked at thus far are shared by humans and animals alike. Like us, animals need to use their bodies, reproduce, move freely in an environment they feel a part of, live as a meaningful part of a group, and feel safe within a territory.

The need for spirituality is unique to humans. But it was also present in the form of man that preceded us, the Neanderthals. We know that Neanderthals buried their dead and decorated the departed, placing at their sides objects that they loved while living. For prehistorians, this fact alone proves that these creatures had a sense of the sacred. Their approach to burial shows that the Neanderthals had a spirituality that rejected death; they saw it instead as merely the passage to another life.

No matter how far back we look, there is no group, society, or civilization that has lived without looking toward the heavens. Each has expressed spirituality in its own way, such as through totems, magic, ancestor worship, fascination with natural forces, petitions to gods, a search for superhuman powers, the search for the absolute, or rites and myths.

Why is this urge so ubiquitous in humans?

Between the last of the apes and the first humans, a crucial event took place: the appearance of self-consciousness. This is not the basic consciousness involved in existing and acting, which other higher animals possess, but something else: the consciousness of being conscious. The event was unprecedented in the evolution of life, and it opened the door to a terrifying reality. Man discovered that his death was inevitable. This revelation represented an unimaginable threat to this new and fragile species. How could people live each day with the certitude that they would one day die?

Pascal wrote a famous meditation on the fear of death. "Imagine a number of men in chains, all under sentence of death, some of whom are each day butchered in the sight of the others; those remaining see their own condition in that of their fellows, and looking at each other with grief and despair, await their turn. This is an image of the human condition."

But as always, evolution found a way to protect our promising species. From the first humans with self-consciousness, evolution selected for survival those whose brains were well-suited to contemplate the irrational and the invisible. This would open up a way to neutralize the terrifying anxiety of our inevitable end.

This is likely how the drive toward the sacred ended up being written into our DNA. Contemplating the spiritual became a way of protecting life. We know that prayer, meditation, and faith produce serotonin and dopamine. The need to believe in something bigger than ourselves helps us to live. That's why a sense of the sacred crossed all cultures, eras, and territories.

In just a few generations, however, that need for the sacred has crumbled under the assault of progress, science, and technology. For a great many, spirituality has all but disappeared. The new idol of consumption has taken the place of the divine.

9. Beauty, wonder, and the aesthetic experience.

How can we explain this need, which no animal seems to experience? What's the reason for the appearance of this intangible attribute, which in a way seems so useless? What good does beauty really do? Why is beauty, like the sacred, written into our programming?

The answer is tied to the previous pillar. The need for the sacred entered our programming when humans were compelled to address the invisible. But our daily language, as profane as it is, was simply inadequate to establish some connection with a god or creator. It seemed inappropriate, even disrespectful.

Thus, to separate ourselves from the profane, another language was born: the language of art. There have been the fantastic cave markings, such as at Lascaux and Altamira, totems, sacred masks, carvings, sculptures, religious music, hieroglyphics, temple decorations, churches, cathedrals, and altar pieces. Art is the manifestation of the beautiful. Although the creation of art is the prerogative of artists, the feeling it produces belongs to every human. That's why for most of history, art has almost always been both religious and anonymous.

It was during the Italian Renaissance that art became secularized, detached from religion. That's when artists first started signing their works. With this gesture, they entered into what would later be called the art market. These were the first hints of consumer society beginning to see the beautiful as merchandise, when previously it was more concerned with utility. It would also give rise to extravagance, scandal, and provocation as a part of the world of art. Marcel Duchamp probably marked the height of this shift, when he exhibited in a museum an upside-down store-bought porcelain urinal, which he signed and titled "Fountain."

Once again, the same forces are at play. They aim to distract us from natural, free sources of satisfaction and to replace them with those that support the economy.

The beautiful is not beautiful in and of itself. We find things beautiful because our brain has been programmed to recognize signals of beauty and then to create reward. The process is the same as with the eight other needs we've looked at. On the surface, aesthetic emotion generates an intense feeling of pleasure. But on a deeper level, it stimulates a discharge of serotonin and dopamine, which recharges the will to live.

10. Consumption and food.

Without this constant and powerful impulse, life wouldn't last more than a few weeks. This need involves powerful pleasures and high levels of rewards. And it's here that consumer culture has found its golden goose.

Food is the ultimate human need that can be exploited and commercialized. Thus, the consumption industry's strategy is the exact opposite of its strategy for other needs. While it usually works by imposing restrictions, for food it opts for exponential increase. This is done through industrial processing to make products more concentrated, and by carefully honing the sensory message attached to products. These all combine to make modern food products as addictive as possible.

The need for food and the need for play both revolve around addiction and profit. Play takes place via television, with its multitude of channels, electronic games that are ever-more addictive, and the Internet and its related devices, which are likely just in their infancy.

Population pressures and the goal of indefinite growth, propelled by constant technological advances, have locked us into the status of consumers. To solidify this status, every effort has been made to diminish natural satisfactions that are immediate and free and replace them with profitable ones in the form of food and games.

This new equation, which runs counter to human nature, creates suffering for which we automatically seek alleviation. We grasp on to anything we can obtain in stores, seeking the satisfaction provided by food and screens.

The reduced scope of our satisfactions leaves us in a compulsive state and results in a constant state of demand. It pushes us to eat too much and to eat badly, and to remain sedentary. That's the basic explanation for how we have become machines for producing excess weight, obesity, and diabetes in just two generations.

Feeding a Deficiency

Now, when I speak with a new patient who has problems with excess weight and diabetes, I systematically ask a number of questions to explore each of the natural sources of fulfillment. Almost every time, I see that their weight gain has developed in conjunction with a decrease in happiness in many of these areas.

The more areas in which we lack satisfaction, the more desperate and inescapable is our compulsion to eat and our willingness to avoid movement by finding distraction in front of a screen.

If a woman tells me that she is widowed or divorced and that her children or grandchildren live far away, there's a good chance she's not finding satisfaction in love, sexuality, and family.

If she is retired, unemployed, or doesn't enjoy her work, she is cut off from another source of fulfillment.

If she doesn't like where she lives, another door is closed.

If she has an urban lifestyle and lacks connection with nature, yet another need is unfulfilled.

If she has ended up in a somewhat solitary life and is sometimes marginalized because she is overweight, she may find herself without a community.

Finally, if the spiritual and aesthetic side of life is absent, everything seems to lead to a choice between two terrible options: depression or obesity.

I don't think I've ever seen anyone who has deficiencies in all of these areas combined. But among those who have gained a lot of weight over a long period of time, I have observed less success in obtaining the simple, natural, and basic satisfactions. My next book, *The Ten Pillars of Happiness,* will explain this fundamental process and also be a source of new ideas on how to understand and reverse the trend.

Chapter 3
The Engine that Drives the Weight Crisis: Sugar and Insulin

As I have explained, this book is aimed at pregnant women today and those who plan on becoming pregnant in the future. As your pregnancy progresses, you will be exposed to a Standard American Diet that has become increasingly artificial over the last 30 years and that contains far too many processed carbohydrates. This new diet may be tolerable for adult women, but the same isn't true for a developing fetus.

An adult pancreas has many functions. What we're most concerned with here is its function as an endocrine gland. The pancreas secretes insulin, among other things. Insulin is a hormone that plays an important role in human physiology. One of its main purposes is to regulate a person's blood glucose level (ideally, in the context of a natural human diet). After each meal containing carbohydrates, the pancreas prevents concentrations of glucose in your blood from reaching levels that would be extremely toxic for all the organs that the blood reaches.

Today, however, the human pancreas is forced to behave differently than it has in the past. That's because it is responding to the invasion of processed foods. If today's diet harms and overworks the adult pancreas, the assault is infinitely more damaging for the nascent pancreas of a fetus developing in its mother's womb.

The window for establishing protection against the new foods that have flooded our diet comes at the end of your third month of pregnancy. That's when the first cells of your fetus's pancreas start preparing to secrete insulin.

What Actually Happens

If you are an adult human female, you have 5 liters of blood in your body. If you are not diabetic, your blood has approximately 1 gram of glucose per liter, when fasting. So, if 1 liter of blood contains 1 gram of glucose, 5 liters contains 5 grams. Based on the total volume of your blood, that equals barely more than a teaspoon of white sugar.

Now, let's imagine a typical situation. You're in a grocery store and buy a box of cookies. You're feeling stressed or rushed, so you open the package. You put one cookie in your mouth, then another. Over the next 15 minutes, you end up eating about a third of the box. It's okay, you tell yourself; you aren't the first to resort to sweet treats to calm yourself down and have a little enjoyment.

Before you throw the package in the garbage, you stop and read the nutritional information. The first line on the rectangular label will probably tell you the number of calories per serving. A serving may be around 100 grams.

Lower down on the label, you'll find the information you should really be after: the total carbohydrates, or the amount of sugars in a serving of the product.

If it's a typical cookie, the amount will be between about 60 to 70 grams per serving, the average being 65 grams of carbohydrates per serving.

So, by consuming that generous helping of cookies, you will have ingested 110 grams of carbohydrates in the form of white flour and sugar. Carbohydrates are among the most invasive sugars; they end up in your blood within half an hour.

With the 5 grams you already had in your blood, this influx ends up raising the total blood sugar level massively: 5 grams + 110 grams = 115 grams.

At the liter level, this would bring your blood glucose level to around 2,300 mg/dl. Any doctor will tell you that no human can survive with a blood sugar level that high: at 1,000 mg/dl, you're at risk of falling into diabetic coma.

But we know from everyday experience that, unless you have severe diabetes, you won't really die from eating a box of cookies. How do we explain this apparent contradiction? The explanation is simple. Since you're not in the final stage of diabetes, your pancreas is able to perform its basic function and control your blood sugar level. Here's what happens, in closer detail.

It all starts in the moment when you decide to buy the cookies and open the package. Your pancreas receives a signal and starts to anticipate what's coming by secreting insulin. Then, as the cookies enter your mouth and start to get digested, the secretion acceler-ates. Finally, when the sugars enter the blood and get converted into glucose, a massive amount of insulin is released to deal with this potentially life-threatening inundation.

Insulin has only limited and poorly adapted means to deal with the situation. It may be starting to seem like a mantra: no pancreas, ani-mal or human, was designed to face foods that are as rich in sugar, as penetrating and invasive, as sucrose (white table sugar), or even worse, today's white flour.

With no natural means of destroying this excess glucose, your body has a different way to counter the problem: flushing it out of the blood. The sugars expelled from the blood end up being stored in three places. These physiological storage facilities are the liver, the muscle, and the adipose tissue.

- The human liver is able to store 50 grams of glucose in a com-pressed form: glycogen. But the liver of today's sedentary human is usually dealing with a backlog of sugar. Still dealing with the sugars that accumulated during the previous meal, it can only absorb a small part of the new sugars coming in.

- The glucose, therefore, tries to rest in the muscles, which nor-mally consume a lot of glucose, storing it in the form of glycogen. But the situation ends up being the same as with the liver. The muscles of the average person today are overloaded with accumu-lated glycogen and can only take in a small portion of the sugar.

- And, so, disturbing amounts of glucose finally head for the adipose, or fatty, tissue. There, they encounter no obstacles. That's because the primary role of the adipose tissue is to store energy in the form of fat: the material designed by evolution to pack a maximum of calories into a minimum of space. Fatty tissue in a human being can easily take in a million calories.

Of course, the reality is much more complex than what I've described, but that, in a nutshell, is the process. Faced with highly toxic quantities of glucose, insulin converts the heavy doses of this nutrient into a substance that's fully tolerated by the organism: fat. It's no exaggeration to say that insulin saves your life by taking on the threat—but it does so at the cost of weight gain that makes you fat.

Insulin has the ability to activate the creation of new adipose cells to further increase fat-storage ability. That means it has the effect of causing weight gain. Indeed, that's not a surprise. We've been aware of the relation between insulin and weight gain since the 1960s.

The science can get complicated, but there's a simple way to frame all this. In the words of Harvard professor George Cahill, "Carbohydrate is driving insulin is driving fat." And since insulin production is triggered by carbohydrate consumption, carbohydrates are primarily to blame for weight gain. This is shown by the direct, chronological correlation between the diabesity crisis and the massive spread of processed foods, rich in invasive carbohydrates, in today's diet.

The biggest factor in the secretion of insulin is the kind of carbohydrate ingested. The type of carbohydrate determines how upset the pancreas will become and how much insulin it will secrete as a result. More specifically, a carbohydrate's power to cause weight gain is determined by the ease with which it will be digested and absorbed.

Above, we looked at the one-off effects of a single package of cookies on an adult pancreas. But what happens if this consumption of invasive carbohydrates occurred on a daily basis? What it leads to is a regular secretion of insulin, and therefore, increasing weight gain.

And this is the situation for the great majority of persons who are overweight or obese or have diabetes.

Imagine the case of an overweight person who, instead of eating meat, fish, and green vegetables, regularly consumes white bread, potatoes, fruit juice, white rice, and cookies, doesn't shy away from beer, and adds two teaspoons of sugar to their coffee. Then there's the next level up: those who drink sugary sodas and eat dips, chips, and candy.

I think that many people, especially those who are experiencing weight problems, would think that this is a pretty normal diet and would admit that it's similar to their own.

After eating this way for some time, varying from person to person according to the amount of sugars being consumed, a phenomenon arises that is truly disastrous for the organism: *insulin resistance*. (Remember the term; it will become as crucial as the term *glycemic index*.)

Insulin Resistance

How does insulin resistance happen? The short answer: too many fast carbohydrates and too little insulin.

Gradually, the body's cells responsible for mopping up excess glucose start being affected by the toxicity of the sugar. Battered and exhausted, unable to do their job, these cells end up resisting the orders they receive from insulin. To compensate for that resistance and ensure your survival, the pancreas must therefore secrete a little more insulin to obtain the same result. But, over time, the resistance increases.

As we've already seen, more insulin equals more weight gain. If the consumption of sugars continues and is not corrected—if it becomes addictive—extra weight quickly becomes obesity.

During all this, the strength or weakness of the person's pancreas becomes a factor. Over time, increased and prolonged exertion by the pancreas can end up wearing out the organ. This leads to two possibilities:

1. If the pancreas is strong and healthy, obesity will take hold and can even worsen; but this will not necessarily lead to diabetes.

2. If, however, the pancreas is vulnerable and fragile, it ends up becoming exhausted and gives up trying to control blood sugar. When this occurs, obesity is associated with diabetes.

But why does this difference exist between one pancreas and another? Why are some strong while others are fragile and vulnerable? If you were already asking yourself this question, I've succeeded in one of my goals, and I'm thrilled to be able to give you an answer: through your dietary choices, you and you alone have the power to determine whether your child will have a strong pancreas or a fragile one.

Only a certain number of obstetricians and diabetologists who focus on gestational diabetes are fully aware of the impact of the maternal diet on the development of a fetal pancreas and the subsequent vulnerability of this pancreas.

Obviously, then, pregnant women are not aware of the facts. How could we expect otherwise? Like all of us, pregnant women are bombarded by flashy, persuasive ads that tell them that there's nutritional value in cookies that are more than 70 percent fast carbohydrates. It took decades for us to succeed in limiting advertising for alcohol and tobacco. Obstetricians have been able to convince their pregnant patients of the importance of avoiding these products. The battle we face now is to do the same for white sugar and white flour.

THE GLYCEMIC INDEX

The glycemic index is a tool that allows us to rate the invasive power of foods containing carbohydrates. This oft-used index measures the ease with which foods containing carbohydrates are digested and assimilated, from their being chewed to their arrival in the bloodstream (it's a little more technical and complicated, but that's it in a nutshell).

This index goes from 0 to 100: 0 is the level of water, and 100 is the level of pure glucose.

The fastest carbohydrate is the ultra-concentrated glucose in your blood. Its glycemic index is 100.

White sugar, or sucrose, is 70—a high number.

All-purpose flour—what you find in bread or cookies —is 85.

Anything below 40 is considered a low number. The medium range lies between 40 and 60, and anything above 60 is considered to be a high glycemic rating.

When a diet puts too many sugars in the body, other related phenomena start to appear. First, persistently high levels of sugar in the blood and in all the organs that it feeds creates oxidative stress, an unmanageable amount of free radicals circulating in the blood. These waste products are the result of glycation, the binding of a sugar molecule and a protein. They're responsible for aging of delicate tissue, the heart, the kidneys, and in particular, the skin of the face.

Being overweight also results in adipose cells growing in size, which alters their functioning. This leads to the production of cytokines, which are vectors of harmful inflammation.

Finally, secreting high levels of insulin exhausts the kidneys, which causes less effective elimination of salt and uric acid. Too much salt in the blood causes water retention and hypertension, and too much uric acid can lead to stones and gout.

What It Means for a Food to Be Refined and Industrially Processed

We've been talking a lot about refined or processed foods. Since industrially produced foods are here to stay, and are even likely to spread, it's important to understand exactly what the terms mean and what they refer to. This knowledge will be especially useful if you're pregnant and eating for two.

Which foods are the ones that are altered and made toxic by the industrial process? From the vast selection of foods available, how do you choose those that are the least processed?

As with our imaginary situation with the package of cookies, the following example of modern-day corn processing will change your entire outlook and permanently alter your approach to food.

The Corn Process: From the Cob to Corn Flakes

Imagine you're walking through a cornfield and you pick off an ear of corn. Later, you grill it and eat it right off the cob. In this fresh and natural form, a grilled cob of corn has a low glycemic index. That's because its strong, dense vegetal texture demands that the body go through a long, exerting process to digest and break down its fibrous matter. The sugars extracted from the chewed and digested grains arrive in the blood gradually, raising blood sugar very moderately. Insulin secretion, therefore, remains weak.

The glycemic index of grilled corn is 36. Based on the overall parameters, that's a relatively low rating.

Now, imagine that a manufacturer decides to package and sell this freshly picked ear of corn in the form of a can of kernels. The manufacturer shells the corn and immerses it in a liquid solution. As the can sits on the shelf, waiting to be sold, the kernels soften as they soak.

This softening of the grain's flesh and skin constitute the equivalent of predigestion. Your body no longer has to do the work, which makes it that much quicker to digest and absorb the corn's sugars. The sugars therefore arrive faster and in greater number, causing a sharper rise in blood sugar and more secretion of insulin as a response.

When it is shelled and soaked in a solution in a can, the same corn picked from the field becomes dangerous and causes weight gain. In this form, the grain's glycemic index rises from 36 to 50.

Now, let's take the scenario a little further. Another manufacturer takes the grains of corn and decides to make flour from them. The grains are dehydrated and very finely ground; they end up in a beige powder form, which can be used for baking or in sauces. This additional processing further erodes the corn's vegetal structure and reduces the effort necessary for digestion.

In the mouth, the stomach, and the small intestine, where the food enters the blood in the form of glucose, digestion and absorption time is reduced, yet again. It leads to an even larger eruption of glucose. Blood sugar jumps even more drastically, forcing the pancreas to increase its production of insulin even further.

When rendered as flour in this form, the glycemic index of corn climbs even higher than before. It reaches close to 70, which is the glycemic index of white sugar.

The final scenario: A third manufacturer takes this flour and makes it into a paste, which is then milled until it's a small fraction of an inch thick. The ultrafine paste is then cooked until it becomes rigid. Finally, it is broken up into the thin pieces we all know under a common name: corn flakes.

When this final transformation is finished, every trace of the original plant has vanished and a nutritional void remains.

When you consume corn flakes, your digestive tract has almost no work to do. The trajectory from mouth to blood becomes a virtual toboggan ride, with no friction along the way. With the arrival of these sugars in the blood, the pancreas secretes almost the largest dose of insulin possible.

What we see when we look at corn flakes, however, is merely another food product: fun, crunchy, and with a charming orange color that's pleasant for kids and reassuring for parents.

And yet the glycemic index of the corn, now processed to the hilt and transmuted into corn flakes, has reached a new peak: between 85 and 92, depending on the country in which it's manufactured.

Remember, we started with a glycemic index of 36 for corn in its most natural form, when it was still in the farmer's hands. We saw this index rise with each step of manufacturing: 50 when it was canned, 70 when it was made into flour, and as high as 92 when it was turned into corn flakes.

I chose the example of corn because it's a shocking one, and because you, and all consumers, should be aware of the effects of the industrial processing of foods. The same process is involved in almost 70 percent of the food we eat. The consequences are serious enough that we should be aware of them, at the very least.

I'm certain that this chain of processing is an integral part of the explosion in weight problems, obesity, and diabetes around the world.

Switching the Blame from Fats to Sugar

The public finally started hearing about the dangers of sugars in the 1970's. The warnings were prompted by scientists who were concerned about the exaggeration and misinformation they saw in the war against fat and cholesterol in the United States. This war had started because of the supposed role of fat and cholesterol in the incidence of cardiovascular disease. And, almost automatically, restriction of fats opened the door wide for the broad carbohydrate family, which includes all sugars.

A Biased Study

The attack on fat and cholesterol, which began in the United States and was spread throughout the media, largely started with Ancel Keys, an ambitious professor at the University of Minnesota. Keys made his reputation with the Seven Countries Study, which he led in 1956. The study showed that countries such as Finland and the United States that consumed large amounts of animal fats also had high rates of heart attack. Countries in southern Europe, however, such as Greece or Italy, that consumed more carbohydrates and vegetable fats, had lower heart attack rates.

It was on this shaky premise that the fierce crusade against cholesterol and high-fat foods began. In order to fill the significant dent that this made in the human diet, a blank check was written for the consumption of carbohydrate-heavy foods. Moreover, this occurred at a crucial moment, when the food industry started gaining access to high technology for processing and refining carbohydrates.

The seven countries had been deliberately selected to get the hoped-for results. Thus, France, the land of cheese, steak, and mayonnaise, was cast aside because its heart attack rate was relatively low. Inversely, Chile was ignored since its heart attack rate was high but its fat consumption was low.

Furthermore, in recent years, many have been asking how a movement of such magnitude could have begun and spread around the world over half a century, when its scientific foundation was so questionable and its claims had such far-reaching consequences. Many point to the power of the lobbyists for the sugar and pharmaceutical industry; the former profit directly from the enormous sugar industry, and the second profits from diseases that result from sugar consumption.

But, whatever the reason, at the time, this study, which had a massive impact on the public, was supported and promoted by the media, politicians, and scientific authorities. The majority of America's nutritionists followed suit.

In 1961, Keys received the support of the American Heart Association, the country's leading scientific body. Their endorsement gave him unshakable authority and earned him the nickname "Mr. Cholesterol." Things went so far during that time that shoppers were offered blood tests for cholesterol in supermarkets in the United States.

John Yudkin's Sugar Scandal

In 1972, in the midst of this fervor, John Yudkin, professor of nutrition at the University of London, published *Pure White and Deadly*.

This book, which came from a recognized authority, created a scandal. It directly contradicted Keys' position. The sugar industry got involved, contradicting his carefully developed theory. Yudkin was forced to use every tool he had to stand up to what he saw as a threat to his integrity. He was opposing an industry that until that time had exercised its power without meeting any resistance.

Yudkin was personally attacked and portrayed as a fanatic; his ideas were dismissed as "emotional assertions." As a result of the media lynching, he was discredited and marginalized by the scientific community. He found himself unable to publish. As all this was transpiring, the sugar industry was funding studies to show that sugars are benign, bolstering their claim with relentless advertising and the creation of ever more addictive and seductive products.

When Yudkin died, he was defeated and forgotten.

Robert Atkins Enters the Fray

In 1972, cardiologist Robert Atkins published *Dr. Atkins' New Diet Revolution,* a book that became an international bestseller. His weight-loss method differed from Keys' in every way. It was based on drastic reduction of all carbohydrates and removed all limits on fats. After an intense wave of success, Atkins became subject to attacks as virulent as those Yudkin had faced.

Twenty years later, many doctors and nutritionists recognized that Atkins had been correct—Atkins had been correct. Research shows that people on a low-carbohydrate diet lose weight more easily than people who follow other diets. Walter Willett, head of the world's leading nutrition research center, Harvard School of Public Health, believes that Atkins was unfairly targeted.

David Jenkins Introduces the Glycemic Index

In 1980, professor David Jenkins created and began promoting the concept of the glycemic index, which would become a major tool in the prevention of diabetes and weight problems. As previously mentioned, this index measures food absorption and the impact of that absorption on blood glucose concentrations and insulin secretion. The major advantage of this index is that it used provable facts and numbers to show the degree of toxicity of a carbohydrate-containing food.

By insisting that sugar is one of the most penetrating and dangerous carbohydrates, Jenkins, too, came under heavy fire, drawing criticism and unconcealed hostility from lobbyists. Today, he says, "I see myself as someone who has always been under the heat of controversy because the concepts I introduced were new to their times."

Today, the glycemic index concept is an undeniable scientific fact. It gives us a simple way to show the impact of different foods on the pancreas. Now that the entire international community is deeply concerned with the weight and diabetes epidemic and wants to find a solution, the nutritional labels on food packaging are poised to be the primary tool to protect consumers and the public.

Picture yourself shopping in a supermarket. As you walk down the aisle, you decide to bring a smile to the face of your young child, and you grab up a box of cereal from the shelf. Television commercials have told you that the cereal, served with milk, is an ideal healthy meal for your child. But as you're about to put the colorful box into your cart, something catches your eye: a bright red warning showing the cereal's glycemic index level. You take a closer look. The glycemic index is 80—higher than white sugar.

Today, however, this labeling, which would do so much to protect the consumer, is prohibited. It's nothing short of an outrage.

Michel Montignac's New Weight-Loss Method

Basing his work on Jenkins' discoveries, Michel Montignac made waves in the '90s by offering a new weight-loss method. Like Jenkins, Montignac recommended excluding sugars, and, by extension, the carbohydrates with the highest glycemic indexes, from one's diet. And, like Jenkins, Montignac faced fierce attacks from lobbyists, which used the fact that he wasn't a doctor as extra ammunition.

The sugar and white flour industries wield enormous hidden power on our political decision-makers, the media, advertising agencies, the medical community, and the general public.

The smear campaigns mentioned above aren't their only tactic. The industry has mastered a carefully constructed strategy of misinformation. The strategy boils down to this: create maximum promotion for sugary and floury products, and put out effective counter-advertising for any and all who point out the dangers.

One of their most effective methods is to try to draw attention away from the most effective weapon against obesity and diabetes: diet. The mouthpieces for this attack are often psychologists, doctors, consultants paid for by the biggest brands in the sugar industry, associations looking for sponsors, and researchers angling to receive funding. For them, diet is something of an easy target. They may talk about the unbearable trauma that a diet can bring.

But we also see another approach: Ineffective diets are endorsed, while truly effective diets, which represent a financial threat, are criticized. The most glaring example of this is that we continue to see diets based on calorie counting, even after 50 years of failure. The only explanation for the continued popularity of these diets, which we are finally realizing are counterproductive, is that the processed food industry has persistently supported them.

Dieting under Fire

The calorie-based concept of diet is actually based on a dogmatic assertion: "All calories are equal, regardless of their origin." Every doctor knows that this claim is false. But repeated often enough, a mistruth becomes accepted as fact.

For 50 years, it had been held as true—against the evidence—that 100 calories from fish is equal to 100 calories from sugar. Why did the doctors who supported that view ignore the fact that diabetes develops because of sugar's toxicity, and not because of calories? Why did they overlook the fact that 80 percent of diabetics are overweight, and that insulin controls sugar by turning it into fat?

But today, the dogma of calories, which paralyzed the fight against invasive sugars and the weight crisis, is finally starting to be discredited. Health authorities are being forced to take responsibility, and, facing pressure from the World Health Organization, are starting to change their position. But, unfortunately, this change doesn't equal victory. The calorie dogma is being replaced with an ever-more insidious view. Since the calorie dogma is untenable, our attention is being drawn away from diets altogether. The message: diets are useless.

Hence, a leading voice in the US launched a campaign that has become ubiquitous in France: stop dieting. Commentators with no medical training rushed to support the trend. Coaches, bloggers, and more claimed to have lost dozens of pounds without having given up any foods.

Then there's the argument put forward by various psychologists who have suggested that watching your diet is equivalent to abuse, a kind of cognitive restriction. Some have even described dieting as orthorexia nervosa, a condition that can lead to severe consequences for mental health. These voices tell us that all you need to do to lose weight is listen to your feelings, to make a distinction between craving and hunger, or, better still, to simply accept your weight.

When you need to lose weight but you lack the necessary motivation, it's comforting to hear that dieting only leads to frustration and unpreventable binge-eating that is actually the sole cause of the weight and obesity crisis. Sugar lobbyists have so much power that they can tell the world—without fear of ridicule—that two billion overweight people and half a billion diabetics are *victims of their own attempts to lose weight*. And then there's the 20 percent of people who have lost weight and still haven't regained it five years later—a group that this view conveniently fails to account for.

An even more sophisticated stratagem emerged a few years ago: the concept of balance. To lose weight, all you need to do is have a balanced diet that consists of a bit of everything, in moderation.

Who could oppose a concept as noble and pure as balance? However, those who have helped obese people lose weight and who know what these people go through are aware that we don't gain weight by choosing the wrong foods; we get bigger because we make choices that are rooted in our pain and ignore whether the foods are fattening. The word "compulsive" is the key here. Those who are prone to compulsive behavior suffer from being overweight; but, they suffer even more if they deny themselves the foods that cause weight gain.

Eating in a balanced way is healthy and worthwhile. Such a diet no doubt makes it possible to stabilize your weight, but it in no way helps you *lose* weight. As a solution for obese people, it's simply not the answer.

Link between Sugar and Toxicity Gains Credit

For five years now, the leading voices in the scientific community in the United States—the country with the highest obesity and diabetes rates—have been warning us about the dangers of sugar.

One of these voices belongs to Robert Lustig, professor of pediatric endocrinology at the University of California. Lustig has probably done more work than anyone else today on sugar and fructose. He considers them poisons. "Sugar," he said, "is the biggest culprit of the country's explosive rate of obesity. Sugar has poisoned food and disrupted people's biology."

Lobbyists continue to oppose Lustig's claims and struggle to reduce the impact of his work. But it's becoming harder for them to hide the seriousness of the health epidemic in the United States, or the soaring numbers of child and adolescent diabetes cases. Lustig's reputation, his position in the scientific community, and his charisma and ability to inspire trust has given him a degree of immunity that Yudkin, Atkins, and Montignac lacked. Lustig has the courage to tell us, "The food industry has its hands free to put any amount of sugar in any food it wants. That is the problem."

Lustig is aiming at more than just obesity and diabetes. He considers these to be elements of the broader issue of metabolic syndrome. His focus as a pediatrician is on the tragic effects of our modern-day diet on human beings at an extremely young age. In his view, sugar and fructose are alcohol for children; in the same way that alcohol can destroy an alcoholic's cirrhotic liver, sugar is capable of profoundly altering the liver's functioning and structure.

Metabolic syndrome is affecting growing numbers of children today. This is known to lead to abdominal weight (belly fat), hypertension, high cholesterol, high triglycerides, fatty liver, and diabetes. And Lustig predicts that when today's children reach adulthood, they will face frighteningly widespread levels of heart attacks.

Very recently, he conducted a study on the effects of hidden sugars on this metabolic disorder, which is affecting children in such large numbers. For this study, his team selected obese children who consumed too much added sugar and fructose and who had high blood pressure, high fasting blood glucose levels, high insulin levels, and elevated liver enzymes, along with obesity. The diet developed for these children reduced or replaced sugars from fruits, grains, bread, and pasta, but without changing the number of calories they take in.

After only nine days on this diet, the benefits were remarkable. All the parameters improved, without any weight loss whatsoever. Blood pressure dropped, blood glucose and insulin levels dropped, triglycerides plummeted, bad cholesterol dropped, good cholesterol rose, the liver reduced in size, and biological markers improved.

What this study confirms is that all calories are *not* equal, and that only those with added sugars are responsible for metabolic disorders leading to diabetes, obesity, and fatty liver.

The subject is complex, but Lustig's demonstration is shockingly clear. I strongly recommend watching *Sugar: The Bitter Truth*, a documentary that has received six million views on YouTube since it was released in 2009. The lesson of the documentary can be summed up in five words: beware of sugar and fructose.

As a pediatrician, Lustig believes that the younger the child, the more dangerous their exposure to sugar and fructose and the greater the necessity for prevention. Lustig and I are allies in this respect.

Chapter 4

Development of the Pancreas in the Embryo and Fetus

In just 30 years, our modern diet has resulted in two generations of newborns that are born larger than previous generations and that are afflicted with a latent vulnerability. This vulnerability is the cause for a two-pronged crisis: excess weight and diabetes. That's my theory; now it's time to prove it. The key piece of evidence is the pancreas, your own, but especially that of your unborn child, which is absolutely more sensitive and vulnerable.

The role of the pancreas is to monitor and regulate blood glucose levels. When this rate exceeds 140 mg/dl, there are risks to the eyes, heart, kidneys, brain, and arteries of the lower limbs. To prevent these problems, the pancreas reacts by secreting insulin, which lowers the glucose level to around 100 mg/dl, where it is perfectly tolerated. The pancreas and its insulin arsenal play this role throughout a person's life.

Up until the 1960s, processed foods containing carbohydrates were rarely encountered under normal living conditions. Pregnant women consumed very little of them; human infants were born weighing about 6.6 pounds and had a normal pancreas.

When a pregnant woman today eats modern foods (as the rest of us do), the pancreas of the fetus she carries will have to deal with the excess glucose in their shared blood *much too early*. A healthy adult's pancreas may be able to tolerate an aggressive diet; the same isn't true of the pancreas of a developing fetus. Facing an environment saturated in sugar, this small pancreas will experience the following:

- Higher than normal birth weight. The child will be born bigger, and its pancreas will be bigger as well, having been forced to work too hard and too soon.

- Vulnerability to weight problems and diabetes. This child will have a persistent tendency to have excess weight during a lifetime, starting at birth, in childhood or adolescence, or later.

- Early appearance of a progressive loss of insulin sensitivity, known as insulin resistance.

Let's say the child is female, and let's follow her further. When this girl has grown up, she is likely to be overweight. Let's say she gets pregnant. During her pregnancy, she will transmit that same pancreatic vulnerability to her fetus. If that fetus faces a nutritional environment as overwhelmed by carbohydrates and processed foods as her mother's when she was in the womb, her child will be born with vulnerability that has only been compounded by the repetition of the cycle.

The idea here is that of the harmful effects of processed carbohydrates on the development of the fetal pancreas are *transmitted and amplified with each new generation*. This domino effect of the weakening of the pancreas makes its victims more prone to weight gain and diabetes. This transgenerational cycle is the cause of the meteoric rise in weight problems.

But here's another shocking thing: it's very easy to stop this escalation. There is one particular moment when the conflict between our ancient pancreas and the sugars of today is most acute and has the most drastic consequences. This is the moment when the pancreas starts to form in the fetus's abdomen.

During those important 60 days, months four and five of your pregnancy, when the pancreas of your fetus is appearing and developing, consume as many natural foods and as few processed carbohydrates as possible by following the plan in Chapter 5 of this book. If maternal nutrition is balanced and moderate, and invasive sugars are limited during this crucial period, the fetal pancreas will develop as it should according to the genetic conditions of our species. That means the pancreas stands a good chance of being robust enough to deal with these foods.

If, however, the fetal pancreas appears in an environment filled with carbohydrates and is permeated with maternal blood that often has high levels of glucose, this pancreas will have gotten off to a bad start; it will be impaired. This pancreas will have a continuing tendency for insulin hypersecretion, and the child will be likely to have a higher birth weight than average, a predisposition for insulin resistance, and a propensity for obesity and diabetes.

The Epigenetics Revolution

Thirty years ago, Dr. David Barker, a British epidemiologist, found extensive evidence that the children of malnourished mothers have below-average birth weight. It was the first time that a link had been found between an event in early life, birth weight, and a health risk that affects adults. His fundamental observation was that during pregnancy, the fetus can be affected in a way that will change its birth weight and leave it with a lifelong vulnerability to certain diseases in adulthood.

Dr. Jennie Brand-Miller, a specialist in infant nutrition and a world authority on the effects of carbohydrates on children's health:

Maternal nutrition is more important than we ever imagined. Life inside the womb is a critical period for metabolic programming that influences a baby's cell types, cell numbers, body composition, hormonal feedback, metabolic activity, and appetite. Our food supply and dietary recommendations should be based first and foremost on the needs of pregnant women. If we cover them, we automatically cover everyone else. They should not be seen as the exception to the rule and simply be given nutritional supplements. We now also know that different patterns of growth have long-term effects on the risk of specific diseases. If growth is restricted, there is a higher risk of abdominal obesity, cardiovascular disease, and type 2 diabetes as an adult. Over-nutrition, seen for example in maternal diabetes and obesity, is also linked to increased risk of obesity in adult life. The positive news is that we know that interventions in pregnancy are probably more effective than later interventions. So we have to give Mum and her unborn baby much greater focus.

A new branch of science was born, a powerful and incisive discipline that we now know as epigenetics, the study of how genes are expressed. Since then, researchers have been pouring into this field to explain the origin of some of the most widespread diseases.

Professor Chittaranjan Yajnik, a leading expert in diabetes research, found that at one time the number of malnourished people in India far exceeded the well-nourished and vastly outnumbered the overweight. Today, however, the situation has reversed itself. The country faces a high susceptibility to obesity and diabetes. Yajnik broke down the proportion of what he calls "the thin and fat." His conclusion? Pancreatic vulnerability is acquired in utero, both through malnutrition and over-nutrition.

Today, the Western world no longer suffers from hunger, and industrially processed food has flooded our diet and situated itself into our nutritional model. And for the past 10 years, most developing countries have gone in the same direction. In these countries, there's a strong correlation between poverty and excess weight. The explanation for this relationship is simple: carbohydrates are the least expensive of the three nutrients to manufacture and the only one that causes insulin secretion.

A growing number of studies and research—some focusing on animals, most being epidemiological studies on humans—have confirmed that the maternal diet and a woman's psychological and emotional environment during pregnancy can increase the risk of her child developing a susceptibility to one of the many chronic illnesses that are a byproduct of modern civilization.

Genetics

Before epigenetics was discovered, genetics reigned supreme. There was no competition.

Genetics is the study of genes. The genome is made up of DNA, which is shaped like a double helix. A single DNA sequence contains a virtual library of information. Darwin's theory of evolution centers on the occurrence of small transcription errors in the genome that are passed on from one generation to the next. The errors result in random mutations. These mutations are passed on only if they proved beneficial for the next generation.

In 2011, a major international study, led by Professor Keith Godfrey from the University of Southampton, showed that during pregnancy, the mother's diet can modify the unfolding of the genetic program which steers the infant's development. "We have shown for the first time that susceptibility to obesity cannot simply be attributed to the combination of our genes and our lifestyle, but can be triggered by influences on a baby's development in the womb, including what the mother ate. A mother's nutrition while pregnant can cause important epigenetic changes that contribute to her offspring's risk of obesity during childhood."

The study showed that epigenetic changes observed at birth significantly predicted obesity in early childhood, from six to nine years old.

Of course, this evolution usually takes place over hundreds of millions of years. The process can't adapt to the sudden and frequent changes we face in our chaotically shifting world today.

But, incredibly, it's been discovered that some genetic evolutionary changes have occurred over *just one generation*—changes that would normally take more than one hundred generations to develop.

This contradicted the dogmatic belief that acquired traits can't be transmitted. To our great surprise, we have found that events and environmental pressures can in fact modify how genes function.

Understanding Epigenetics

Genes are almost unalterable; they change only through profound and stable mutations. Epigenetics focuses on the modulation of the *action* of these genes, but not modification of the *sequence*.

Let's consider a simple example of epigenetics at work. All bees in a hive start their life as larvae. But some will end up becoming workers, others will become guards, others will be foragers, and just one will be queen. It all depends on how they are fed.

Here's an even clearer demonstration of what distinguishes epigenetics from genetics. A turtle egg will become a male or female adult turtle *based solely on water temperature*; that's epigenetics at work.

These examples show us that while genes carry a message, the environment can cause *modifications* to that message, to adapt it to the needs of the species. While genes are the motor, the epigenome is the rudder (or the shock absorbers).

We could also think about epigenetics in terms of a symphony by Mozart. The majestic piece of music is mapped out by the composer's hand; eventually it becomes a part of our species' heritage. But in the years that follow, any performer or conductor can bring their own sensibility to the piece, adapting it to the aesthetics of their own time and place. The audience brings their own context to the experience, too, interpreting the music in their own way.

In the broadest terms, then, that's what epigenetics is and how it occurs. Thousands of researchers have been studying this fascinating branch of science, and they've shared their findings with the world.

So, why do you need to know about it?

From the moment your oocyte detaches from your ovary and encounters a man's spermatozoa, an egg is formed. It will divide and redivide 56 times in the process of becoming a child.

As these 56 divisions unfold, epigenetics can intervene to amplify or weaken the unfolding of the genetic message, if the environment demands it. And the role of epigenetics doesn't stop when a child is born; it develops throughout his or her life, following the same principles.

Here's a simplified explanation of how epigenetic effects occur.

Your DNA contains your design. The plan for how you'll operate is inscribed on a double helix coded with just four letters, A, G, C, and T. These are the nitrogenous bases: adenine, guanine, cytosine, and thymine. To intervene on this fundamental text and make modifications, epigenetics uses two methods: DNA methylation and histone modification.

DNA Methylation

In very simple terms, a molecule is methylated when a small appendage is added that modifies its shape. This appendage, which plays a role in epigenetics, is known in chemistry as methyl radical.

For example, let's take cytosine, one of the four base types of the genetic alphabet, and follow it through transcription:

Like all molecules, cytosine's activity is determined by its shape, the same way the shape of a key determines which door it can open. To alter the activity of cytosine, epigenetics modifies the molecule's shape by adding a methyl radical in a specific place that will change the molecule's message.

This task is carried out by an enzyme, methyl transferase, which dislodges the cytosine hydrogen molecule on its fifth summit and replaces it with a CH3 methyl radical.

You might be surprised that such a small change can affect the relay of information. But it can, and the same goes for all types of communication. Think about what would happen if you called your mother on the phone and asked for "Tom" instead of "Mom." All it takes is one single syllable to completely derail the original message.

Histone Modification

The center of operations is the cell. Inside the cell is the nucleus. Inside the nucleus are chromosomes. Each chromosome contains a DNA double helix, coiled around a spool of histones to form a nucleosome. Groups of nucleosomes form chromatin, the raw material of chromosomes. The spool of histones is what gives DNA its density and structure. By changing this density—by increasing or reducing the amount of histones—the genetic message can be modified.

Anatomically, the histone has a tail that extends outside of the nucleosome. Epigenetic changes are made to the histone tail in order to affect the relay of information. There are four different types of histone modifications, but acetylation and methylation occur most frequently. Acetylation is used to promote gene expression, while methylation is used to repress it. Just as a piano's notes can resonate loudly or softly depending on how it is played, genes can either be intensified or muffled.

By combining methylation and histone modification, we arrive at epigenetic modulation of the genetic code within the nuclei of the cells.

Development of the Pancreas

Pregnancy is intricately mapped out. It's akin to a musical score that has been read and interpreted for hundreds of millions of years. The formation of the pancreas is like a single bar on that musical score.

That means that the pregnancy process for a Cro-Magnon woman 40,000 years ago was identical in every way to that of a woman today.

Each week brings changes to the embryo and then to the fetus, all leading to birth. The role and functions of the pancreas, too, were laid out at our origin some 200,000 years ago and remain the same today. And that means that as the pancreas of your unborn child develops, it will follow exactly the same blueprint as the pancreas of an infant caveman ages ago.

The tension between the ancient pancreas and the modern diet is at its height and is most dangerous when this organ first appears. When a pregnant woman relies on processed carbohydrates or refined sugars in her diet, it marks a major event in the 56 divisions of the genetic program that guides the transformation of an egg into a newborn over the course of nine months.

By carefully selecting the right foods to consume during your pregnancy, you hold the power to control that tension. But if you fail to do so, you may make the collision between ancient and modern that much more damaging.

We know that genetics governs our physiology. It may be easier to understand the urgency of protecting the pancreas at the moment when it is formed in the mother's womb by summarizing that formation.

- By the nineteenth day, two small buds appear on the wall of the intestine: first the dorsal bud, and three days later, the ventral bud.

- By the fifth week, these two buds start to migrate so they can meet and merge.

- In the sixth week, the ventral moves toward the dorsal bud, passing underneath and behind it.

- In the seventh week, the two buds have collapsed and merged. At this point, the pancreas is not yet affected by what the mother eats and is incapable of reacting to the foods. The organ is well into its development, but it still lacks the critical ability to secrete insulin. Ninety-nine percent of the developing cells in this pancreas-to-be will eventually play a role in the organ's endocrine function and will produce digestive enzymes; the remaining one percent will be involved in the endocrine function only, with half of them specializing in insulin secretion.

- During the fourth and fifth month, the cells that have so far been undifferentiated will come together into little islets called

Langerhans. Over these 60 days, these Langerhans disseminate and acquire the capacity to secrete insulin. And that's the way it's been for 200,000 years.

While the fetal pancreas forms that ability to secrete insulin, it meets a powerful adversary: excess glucose. The sugars the mother consumes are digested and then broken down so they can end up in the blood in the form of glucose. Glucose is a small molecule, so it easily passes through the placenta, transferring from the mother's blood to that of the fetus. But maternal insulin is too big to pass through the same way. That means the fetus must produce its own insulin.

If the mother consumes products that are high in sugars, her blood sugar level will rise. The fetal pancreas will therefore be required to transform this glucose into fat. This leads to weight gain that is proportional to the sugar consumption, and to increased infant birth weight.

Imagine an everyday situation: An expectant mother prepares a plate of white rice and a glass of fruit juice, or picks up a little sandwich on white bread from the supermarket. In the mother's blood, glucose levels can easily rise to 140 mg/dl. This blood travels to the fetus, which has started developing insulin-secreting cells. However, the small fetal pancreas doesn't have enough insulin to neutralize the sudden influx of sugar. Because the fetus is still developing, it reacts by producing more insulin-secreting cells so it can release a sufficient amount of the hormone. The resulting increase in insulin transforms the sugar into fat and causes the fetus to grow. This causes a higher birth weight. This disturbing phenomenon has been happening regularly for two generations now.

And here's the crux of the problem: Over time, your child's pancreas will continue to hyper-secrete. This makes him or her predisposed to excess weight, insulin resistance, diabetes, and metabolic syndrome. And as we have seen, these pathologies have grown exponentially in the past decade.

By the end of the fifth month, the die is cast. The cells within the Langerhans islets that are responsible for insulin secretion have become functional. Their development, and their eventual strength or weakness, depends on the levels of glucose in the maternal blood that reaches the fetus and its pancreas.

Finally, from the sixth to the ninth month, the volume of the insulin-secreting cells will increase, as well as their insulin production.

To summarize, during the two months of the cellular proliferation phase, or months four and five of pregnancy, the beta cells of the pancreas have more power to multiply than ever, and it's during these two months that maternal nutrition must be regulated most carefully.

PANCREAS WEIGHT GROWTH (third trimester)

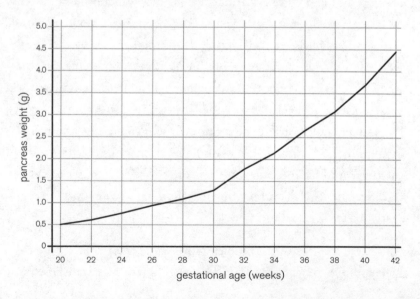

Chapter 5
The Plan

Losing weight is neither simple nor easy, and its process can often be inconsistent. I've designed and created this plan to help stop the obesity and diabetes epidemic by approaching it from a new starting point: just when it's beginning to form. This decisive moment is the time when the pancreas of the fetus begins to emerge and develop in the mother's womb. This approach applies epigenetics to solve the weight crisis here and now.

There are three reasons this program will succeed:

1. It is simple.

2. It is logical.

3. It centers on your most important job during pregnancy: maintaining a good, healthy diet.

You are the only one who can take action and help prevent the pathologies of excess weight, obesity, and diabetes by choosing your diet wisely during the course of your pregnancy, particularly the 60 days of months four and five. The three-phase protection plan in this book follows your pregnancy calendar and varies according to the level of risk for each period.

1. The first trimester. The pancreas is not secreting any insulin, and your diet has some flexibility.

2. The fourth and fifth months. The pancreas begins to secrete insulin. Emphasis will be on this phase, when risk is at its highest. If you watch your diet with extreme care, the benefits will be huge.

3. The final four months of pregnancy. The risk decreases somewhat, and your diet regains a bit of flexibility.

How the Plan Works

The vast majority of women today know that drinking soda and eating corn flakes and candy bars is less healthy than eating a salmon fillet with asparagus. But a great many women still indulge in the less healthy option; after all, it won't kill you. I want to be very clear that this plan is not intended to help you cut calories, and even less to help you lose weight. Its aim is to help you reduce your consumption of certain foods that may disturb the immediate development of the fetus.

The food industries may be able to fool a great many consumers who are unable to see through the fog of misinformation—but it's more difficult to fool a mother-to-be who carries a child in her womb.

The message here is simple and clear: Avoid consuming too many processed carbohydrates. These foods excessively raise the level of glucose in the maternal blood, which reaches the fetus through the placenta.

After a balanced meal consisting of an appetizer, main course, and dessert, your blood sugar can reach 140 mg/dl. If the meal is rich in invasive carbohydrates, your blood sugar can climb even higher. It will climb higher still if you indulge in snacks that are high in sugars, such as a muffin on your way to the office.

Another important point: It's commonly believed that there are two families of carbohydrates, invasive (fast) carbohydrates and gradual (slow) carbohydrates. The difference is thought to be based on their chemical structure and their glycemic index, or the number associated with a particular type of food, indicating that food's effect on blood sugar levels. Remember, the index goes from 1 to 100, with fast carbs, such as flour, being anything above 60, and slow carbs being anything below 40.

Health organizations are finally calling for moderation in the consumption of carbohydrates with a high glycemic index, such as white sugar, white flour, and all their derivatives. They also consider slow carbohydrates to be good foods and recommend consuming starches at every meal, even for diabetics.

Warning: If distinguishing among carbohydrates based on invasive power is valid, it's qualitative and not quantitative. In other words, it doesn't account for the *portion* consumed. In fact, it all comes down to the dose.

Consider the Glycemic Load of Foods

The glycemic index is only helpful if we compare equal quantities of carbohydrates. Let's consider the example of legumes, one of the foods that's lowest on the glycemic index.

When you consume 100 grams of lentils, digestion and absorption is slow and uneven, which raises your blood sugar only moderately. The effect on the pancreas and its secretion of insulin is therefore weak.

If you consume 300 grams of lentils, carbohydrates still arrive in your blood slowly, but in a more concentrated way. Appearing all at once, they have a stronger impact on your blood glucose. The *quantity* alters the situation.

Because of this, we need to take another, more complex index into account: the glycemic load.

Here's how the glycemic load is calculated for a particular food.

Glycemic load = [Glycemic index x quantity of carbohydrates per portion of food (grams)]/ 100

Let's break that down:

1. Start by determining the quantity of carbohydrates in the portion you're investigating. Be careful: don't mistake the amount of carbohydrates for the weight of the food that contains them. One hundred grams of cookies, for example, may contain 45 grams of carbohydrates, or 65, or 70. Check the nutritional labeling carefully.

2. Multiply the quantity of carbohydrates by the glycemic index (between 0 and 100).

3. Divide the product by 100.

What can you learn from the result? Let's see together.

Example: 100 grams of French bread

In 100 grams of French bread, there are 50 grams of carbohydrates.

The glycemic index is 80.

50 x 80 = 4000

Glycemic load = 4000 / 100 = 40

Example: 300 grams of tomatoes

In 300 grams of tomatoes, there are 13.8 grams of carbohydrates.

The glycemic index is 35.

13.8 x 35 = 483

Glycemic load = 483 / 100 = 4.83

HOW TO CLASSIFY GLYCEMIC LOADS	
10 or under	low glycemic load
11 to 19	moderate glycemic load
Over 20	high glycemic load

Examples of glycemic load:

200 grams of cooked couscous: 31.2

200 grams of spaghetti: 35

20 gummy bears: 29

As you can see, 200 grams of couscous or spaghetti has the same effect or higher as 20 gummy bears.

Conclusion: While you may hear that you're supposed to eat starchy foods with each meal, pay close attention to the quantities you eat. Remember that all carbohydrates, from honey to lettuce and white bread to green beans, end up in the blood sooner or later in the form of glucose.

To put it another way, don't make the common mistake of thinking, "If the glycemic index of this food is low, I can eat as much as I want, whenever I want." Don't rely solely on the glycemic index, especially during pregnancy. Consider the quantity as well.

The Three Periods of Pregnancy

The next section consists of a three-phase protection plan based on three distinct periods of your pregnancy, with dietary suggestions for each period.

The First Trimester: Months 1, 2, and 3 of Your Pregnancy

There's one principle that your obstetrician would surely agree with: avoid gaining too much weight at the start of your pregnancy, especially if you're overweight to begin with. During the first trimester of your pregnancy, your baby doesn't have a functional pancreas and is unable to secrete insulin. Follow these guidelines at this stage:

- Follow the Your Daily Diet in Five Basic Steps, below, specifically designed for the fourth and fifth months of pregnancy but recommended for the duration of pregnancy.

- Follow the advice that your doctor gives you.

- Quit smoking and abstain from alcohol.

- Walk for half an hour a day.

- Try to avoid stress. Weigh your daily stresses against the wondrous event of your pregnancy. Don't let insignificant worries threaten your well-being.

- Use this time to prepare for what comes next.

Your Daily Diet in Five Basic Steps

Because these steps are as important as they are simple, I suggest you follow them throughout your pregnancy, from the first day to the last and beyond than that, if you're breastfeeding. I suspect you'll find them so easy, and the results so positive, that you'll end up following them for the rest of your life.

This sense of assurance comes partly from my own life. I've adopted these basic principles for myself. My family has, too. I try to share them with everyone who's close to me, and with anyone who cares about the health and well-being of themselves and their family.

1. Switch from white sugar (sucrose) to coconut sugar. International health guidelines clearly state that sweeteners are allowed. Only pure sugars are responsible for the double epidemic of obesity and diabetes that has already affected two billion people in the world. However, do your research about other types of sweeteners. A recent study has shown that the more a pregnant woman consumes sweetened sodas, the higher the risk of premature delivery, a relationship that has not been observed with light drinks.

I've already mentioned that a certain line of thought says it's wrong to prohibit any food absolutely, because no food is dangerous in moderation. There may be some truth to this. But for every person who can stop at one square of chocolate or a single cigarette after a meal, there are countless others who are unable to resist the desire to consume further.

Some foods lend themselves better than others to moderation. It's not very often you hear of bulimics overindulging on leeks, for instance. And remember, white sugar shouldn't be considered a food. It's a product that has been intensely condensed, refined, and concentrated. The substance it has become borders on the pharmaceutical. We know—and it's finally starting to be said—that the refining and concentration that takes place during the extraction of sugar allows it to activate reward centers in the brain the same way hard drugs do.

Here's a shocking example. Several years ago, a French researcher was studying rats that were regularly administered cocaine. By the fifteenth day, the rats had developed the habit of going to one corner of their cage for their dose of drugs. Then, a second bottle was introduced in the other corner of the cage. The rats hesitated at first, then tasted a bit of each. In the end, they ended up favoring the new bottle. The contents of this bottle were nothing but water and white sugar. Look for the video online; seeing the rats aggressively feed from the bottle and hearing their desperate sounds will really make you think about the effects of sugar on an adult animal.

2. Switch from white bread to whole grain. By white bread, I mean any bread made with industrially processed white flour. Wheat is a wild grain that was domesticated when humans became sedentary. From the dawn of civilization until the mid-twentieth century, the species of wheat we've used has evolved slowly. Over the last 50 years, however, agriculture has revolutionized the process; we have multiplied the number of crossbreeds and hybrids in order to create more manageable species. Wheat is now the modern cereal that has been most extensively modified by humans.

Industry has pushed the transition even further by subjecting flour to physical and chemical treatments to make an even finer powder that can be sifted. White flour is therefore very poor in fibers, minerals, and vitamins, but it's very rich in starch. Processed white bread made from this flour is a true nutritional void, and the carbohydrates it contains are extremely invasive. Let's recall a powerful fact we saw earlier: the glycemic index for industrially produced white flour and the bread made with it is 80, *higher than that of white sugar itself, which is 70.*

And what about whole wheat bread? If the bread is made industrially, it's often reconstituted; it is white bread to which wheat bran has been added. This artificial recomposition is nothing more than a marketing ploy. It's a blending, not a binding. The combination of flours breaks down during the digestive process. The white flour advances much more rapidly than the wheat; it detaches from the stomach and races toward the small intestine, then enters the bloodstream. This causes a steep rise in blood glucose levels. The bran arrives later, after the battle has taken place. The white flour has already been transformed into glucose, and insulin has been summoned to do its job in response.

The situation is very different for whole grain bread, which contains the entire grain, ground up but with no parts sifted out. The end result is flour made up of particles of flour and bran that are fused naturally and have not been separated. Whole grain flour therefore contains all the grain's fibers, as well as the germ. The latter turns rancid very quickly, which means the artisanal bakers who work with it have to grind it quickly and use it all up each day.

Whole grain bread has an extremely low glycemic index (35 to 40), which means only a moderate amount of work for the pancreas during its ultra-sensitive development phase.

During the fourth and fifth months, treat yourself to organic whole-grain sourdough, prepared the old-fashioned way: slow-fermented with stone-milled flour, kneaded by hand.

3. Switch from white rice to whole grain brown rice. Rice is a cereal grain from Asia that started to spread across the world in the twentieth century. It's now used so widely that we have all the facts on the healthy way to consume it.

During your pregnancy, I recommend you switch from white rice to whole grain brown rice. The reasons are similar to what we saw with wheat. The white rice we see today has been husked and polished to improve its yield and make it more attractive. This process has eliminated much of its antioxidants and all the fibers that slowed down its absorption.

In a recent epidemiological study published in the *British Medical Journal*, a medical team from Harvard reviewed a high number of studies that monitored more than 350,000 people in the United States, China, Australia, and Japan over a long period. They found that eating white rice raised the risk of developing diabetes by 25 percent. The risk was as high as 55 percent for people in Asian countries who consumed large amounts regularly.

If you eat white rice often and in large quantities, it's essential that you switch to whole grain brown rice during those crucial two months. You should stick to a normal-sized bowl. If you're not great at self-restraint, switch to whole grain basmati (it's not easy to find, and it's a bit more expensive than most other kinds).

4. Switch from white pasta to whole grain pasta. There are two typical kinds of wheat used for pasta. Hard wheat is used for dry pasta, and soft wheat is used for fresh pasta and Asian noodles. Hard wheat is more resistant to being broken down during digestion and enters the blood more slowly than soft wheat. Opt for pasta made from hard wheat.

However, whole grain pasta is really your best choice, and for similar reasons. It's made with wheat kernels that still have their outer covering. They're richer in vitamins and minerals, but it's their fiber content that really counts for you because of their ability to stem the invasive power of sugars. The ideal, then, is pasta that is both whole grain and made from hard wheat.

But that's not your only concern. Consider how pasta is cooked as well. Follow the Italians' example and cook it *al dente*. Remember, the general rule is that anything that attacks a food's resistance—in this case, cooking—is a form of predigestion. That means less work that will have to be done during digestion, and faster absorption and more drastic blood glucose elevation.

Don't be fooled into thinking that whole grain pasta is less delicious than white. Many who eat it regularly find it denser and more rustic, with a more satisfying chew. This recommendation isn't aimed at you as an adult unless you're overweight or predisposed to diabetes. It is aimed at your unborn child, whose pancreas needs to be protected as it navigates the most crucial part of its development.

5. Switch from fruit juice to whole fruits. Why? For the same reason again: to avoid the products that industries turn from natural to artificial. Under the pretext of making a food more convenient, practical, and easy to consume, the food industry took natural fruit, squeezed it, and turned it into liquid.

"So what's wrong with that?" The answer is juice isn't food. When you squeeze a fruit, you turn a food that you crunch and chew into a liquid that you drink. Again, the following principle applies: The more you transform a food, the more work there is for your pancreas. And this is for a simple reason. Any food you consume must necessarily be broken down into its basic elements to be able to enter the bloodstream.

There are two ways to do this. You can digest it entirely, or you can eat it already transformed, processed, pressed, or cooked. The more a food is predigested, the faster it moves through you. And if it's a carbohydrate-rich food, it will be transformed into glucose faster and in higher amounts, which requires the secretion of more insulin.

When you squeeze a fruit—an orange, for example—take a look at what gets left in the press: all the fibrous web of the pulp has been separated from the juice. That's work that your body would be doing if you ate fruit the way it comes off the tree.

That's why your job is to replace fruit juice with fresh fruits. And now's a good time to remind yourself of what health organizations have recommended for ages: eat five servings of fruits and vegetables each day. It's hard to argue with such sound advice. However, some ambiguity hides within it. Grouping the two families of food under the same heading implies that fruits and vegetables are interchangeable. That's not exactly true, and it may lead to some bad decisions.

Everything that you find in fruit—vitamins, minerals, and fibers—is found in vegetables as well. But there's a profound difference between the two foods. To summarize it simply: a fruit is like a sugary vegetable.

Let's look at a few examples. An average portion of orange or pineapple contains 4 grams of fructose, peach contains 5 grams, watermelon contains 6 grams, grapes contains 8 grams, and pear contains 10 grams.

There are 0 grams of fructose in spinach, mushrooms, celery, broccoli, and lettuce, and 1 to 2 grams in eggplant, asparagus, cabbage, and tomatoes. Only carrots and beets have higher amounts.

This fructose presence doesn't cause any problems for people with a strong pancreas; it does become a problem, however, for those whose pancreas is vulnerable. This is the case for people with diabetes, who are advised not to eat a lot of fruit.

A study in the *British Medical Journal* used data on 187,000 people who were monitored over a 24-year period. Twelve thousand of them developed type 2 diabetes during that time. In comparing their consumption of whole fruits and fruit juice, they found that replacing three portions of fruit juice with whole fruits reduced the risk of diabetes by 7 percent. The risk decreased by 12 percent when people ate, rather than drank, grapefruit, 14 percent for apples and pears, and to 19 percent for grapes.

It was long believed that fructose, which has higher sweetening power than white sugar, has a lower glycemic index. It was therefore thought to be a good substitute for sugar. We now know that fructose is more dangerous for diabetics than glucose, because the liver transforms it more quickly into fat, raising the level of blood triglycerides and helping pave the way for insulin resistance.

So, what is dangerous for the worn-out pancreas of someone with diabetes is even more risky for the fetus during its path to maturity. The risk becomes greater still during months four and five, those 60 days when the organ is being constructed and each intake of sugar forces a reflex response. When this response is repeated again and again, it marks the organ and affects its development.

If you're able to take make the effort of buying organic fruit, do so, and choose them yourself to avoid bruises. Fruit without bruising has even more vitamins and fiber.

Avoid eating fruit by itself, since it consists almost entirely of carbohydrates. Adding just a small amount of fats and proteins can cut fruit's power to penetrate and limit its impact on the pancreas. A single nut and a spoonful of cottage cheese is enough to slow the digestion and absorption of a slice of pineapple.

Also, always eat your fruit at the end of a meal, and not before it. Why? For the same reason that a Maserati can only drive as fast as a tractor when following one on a highway. It slows down the fruit's digestion.

Also, try to avoid overripe fruit. As fruit matures, its starches are increasingly converted into simple sugars (fructose and glucose). What's more, all fruits are not equal. Always consider the potential action of a given fruit on your blood sugar, and by extension, on your unborn child's pancreas.

Here are some foods ranked in descending order according to their glycemic effect:

10. Dates

9. Parsnips, lychee (canned, without pits)

8. Watermelon, melon, pumpkin, squash

7. Dried raisins, sweet potato, dried figs

6. Apricot, ripe banana, kiwi

5. Chestnuts, melon, papaya, mango, fresh lychee, grapes, pineapple

4. Plums

3. Nectarines, apples, oranges, coconut, fresh figs, peaches, pears, tomatoes, passion fruit, mandarins, clementines

2. Black currants, cherries, strawberries, raspberries, blackberries, blueberries, goji berries, passion fruit, ground cherries

1. Rhubarb, peanuts, pine nuts, almonds, walnuts, cashews, pistachios, hazelnuts, olives

Months 4 and 5 of Your Pregnancy

We've come to the key moment in the plan that lies ahead of you: the 60 days when everything you've looked at so far takes on a heightened importance, when it all fits together and becomes actionable. It's here that your intervention will be most decisive.

During these two months, your baby's pancreas will undergo a rapid metamorphosis, undergoing more transformations than it will during the rest of its lifetime. Its little cells, which had been inactive, undifferentiated, and unspecialized, will acquire the capacity to secrete insulin.

As soon as it gains this capacity, the emerging pancreas is capable of capturing glucose in your shared blood, in real time. And it attempts to respond by secreting the necessary amount of insulin. If your diet contains too many foods with a high glycemic index, you will be forcing the cells of the budding fetal pancreas to work at maximum capacity to manage the excess glucose. This abnormal pressure leads to a weakened pancreas that will no longer be able to operate as it's supposed to.

During these two months, you need to modify your intake of the most aggressive and invasive carbohydrates. Five lists will be included as a guideline of foods to eliminate, avoid, moderate, eat freely, and try to eat more of. In addition to following these lists, continue to follow Your Daily Diet in Five Basic Steps (page 91), and above all, let your instincts guide you.

Your mission is to keep your blood glucose level between 80 and 110 mg/dl. Blood sugar isn't just acceptable at this level—it's essential. Above that, however, it becomes harmful. By limiting your intake of invasive sugars, you'll effectively cap your blood glucose levels. That means you'll avoid creating a vulnerability that will be a danger throughout your child's life.

You've probably noticed that there are women who are lucky enough to find invasive sugars fairly unappealing to begin with. They have no taste for sweets like cookies or candy, and aren't drawn to white bread or white rice. These women inevitably have a normal weight, and neither they nor their children have much need to be protected.

For the countless others who do have an attraction to fast carbs, a choice must be made between the fleeting pleasures of carbohydrates and the extraordinary reward of bringing a healthy child into the world.

For 20 years, obstetricians have asked their patients stop smoking during their pregnancy. Most patients accept, including those who have been unable to quit for their own sake. More recently, the recommendation of abstinence has been extended to alcohol. For some years now, it has not been a question of reducing alcohol intake but of eliminating it completely. My goal (and I'm not alone) is to place dangerous sugars in the same category as alcohol and tobacco, at least for the fourth and fifth months, the most critical months for the development of the fetal pancreas.

Months Four and Five: A 60-Day Action Plan for Eating

The basic objective of this plan is quite specific: protecting the development of your developing child's pancreas. The aim is NOT to make you lose weight. Nothing in the roadmap for these two months can be considered, in any way, a weight-loss diet.

In the lists that follow, I've divided carbohydrates into five categories based on how harmful they are to the infant's pancreas. Note that the foods listed on the following pages are only those that primarily contain carbohydrates. Your baby needs proteins, which are as vital for the development and growth of the fetus as they are for the growth of the child, adolescent, and adult. Additionally, your baby needs lipids and fats, because fats make up the cell membranes of the nervous system. So feel free to eat proteins and fats like meat, fish, eggs, dairy products, oils, oilseeds, nuts, and vegetable proteins like tofu.

List I: High-carbohydrate foods to ELIMINATE during months four and five.

These are ranked in descending order according to their invasive effect on the development of the fetal pancreas.

- **Beer**. This is probably the food that is *least* tolerated by an adult pancreas and infinitely less tolerated by a pancreas that is going through differentiation. Because it's an alcoholic beverage, your doctor has probably prohibited it anyway.

- **Potatoes**.

   * **Instant potato flakes.** In its industrially processed form, this hyper-processed food comes in a pretty package that makes it practical and easy to prepare. It's also one of the most quickly

absorbed solid foods, and therefore, extremely aggressive toward the pancreas.

* **Boiled and peeled potatoes**

* **Baked potatoes**

* **French fries**

* **Chips**

* **Potato gnocchi**

- **Bread**.

  * **Gluten-free white bread.** You may be surprised to hear me go against the raging gluten-free trend. To be clear, this recommendation only concerns pregnancy—specifically, those crucial 60 days. If you don't have a gluten intolerance, neither you nor your child have any reason to fear gluten. Gluten, like protein, slows down the digestion and assimilation of sugars contained in wheat flour. Also, about 10 percent of the proteins have been eliminated from gluten-free bread; it automatically contains more carbohydrates.

  * **Biscotti made with white flour.** The harmful effects of white flour are made worse by the fact that biscotti are cooked twice, which further increases the penetrative power of the flour.

  * **Any ultra-white bread.** The bread crust is a bit more resistant to digestion than the rest of the loaf. For this reason, companies have gone so far as to create a crustless loaf of bread, sliced for sandwiches. *Why?*

  * **Baguettes.** Baguettes are enjoyed around the world, and are a sacred tradition in their country of origin. But, remember, we're only talking about 60 days here. And, after all, isn't pregnancy even more sacred?

* **Boxed cereals.** The many rounds of industrial transformation corn goes through to create cereal flakes make the final product more penetrating. Cereals like corn flakes are the pinnacle of processed food technology; they are transformed to be visually appealing with a pleasant consistency, but at the cost of nutritional value. I'm convinced that this cereal, invented in the United States, has played a role in causing the American obesity epidemic. Its impact is all the greater in that the product targets children and is marketed as a good breakfast choice. With this combination of age group and time of day, the danger from carbohydrates is very high.

  However, not all corn flakes are created equal. Brands with the highest protein and fat content are less aggressive and diabetogenic. As paradoxical as it may seem, corn flakes with chocolate reduces the product's glycemic index, thus reducing its impact on the fetal pancreas. But be wary of corn flakes that are sold as diet products.

* **Cornstarch.** Some cooks use small amounts to thicken sauces, which poses minimal risk. Still, better to wait until the end of the crucial 60 days for the pancreas that's budding within your fetus.

• **Aggressive kinds of rice**.

  * **Fast-cooking rice.** To save time for consumers, rice producers precook rice. This action is essentially physical predigestion; it elevates the penetrating power of the rice's carbohydrates.

  * **Sticky rice.** Usually found in Chinese cooking. If you have the option to choose between sticky or standard white rice during the crucial two months, opt for standard. (You'll find it under the second category of carbohydrates).

* **Puffed rice.** This is rice whose husk was been removed with a combination of strong pressure and water vapor. That makes it fun, easy to eat, and up to three times the volume of the original grain. However, it is digested much faster and has a powerful penetrative power.

In India, where many still suffer from hunger, puffed rice (*pori*) is used as a religious offering. Here as elsewhere, dietary traditions and religion have adapted in tandem to respond to the needs of the public. The religious use of puffed rice led Indians to consume it themselves, and the food became a staple in shortage areas.

Turning rice into puffed rice makes it more profitable, and makes it advantageous for survival. It doesn't increase the calorie count, but it makes it flood into the blood more quickly and in greater quantities. Then, more insulin is needed to transform these sugars into fat. What was a blessing for malnourished Indians has turned into a problem for those who live in a culture of abundance where food has been extensively industrialized.

* **Rice cakes.** The same things are true for rice cakes as for puffed rice. However, they're often organic and presented as a healthy, balanced snack. The opposite is true. Marketers tell you that their light weight (around 8 grams) is linked to *your* light weight (present or future). And always remember that organic doesn't mean a low glycemic risk. A food can be grown under the best, pesticide-free conditions and still be diabetogenic.

• **Cookies made with white flour**. These cookies should be avoided entirely during the sensitive two months. However, this does not mean you have to avoid all cookies.

Cookies are one of the snack industry's main products today. If you buy them, it's important to know how to choose them properly. For this, you only need to consider three criteria: the carbohydrate level, the white sugar level, and the type of grain used.

If it's wheat, the flour used will be white and will be absorbed ultra-quickly in your body. If the flour is whole wheat, it will consist of white flour to which a token amount of wheat bran has been added. The mixture separates in the stomach to become white flour again. If, however, the flour is whole grain wheat or rye, the invasive power is truly slower.

The slowest grain is oat bran, with a glycemic index of 15. That's about five times slower than white flour, which is 80.

Be very careful when you read the packaging on cookies. Don't rely on manufacturer claims that a food product is "part of a balanced diet." Trust only the list of ingredients and the carbohydrate levels on the nutritional label. These two facts mean a lot more than any other kind of health claim.

When you're past your pregnancy, I suggest you keep the habit of going by these three criteria, for yourself and for your family. If a serving of a food has more than 50 grams of carbohydrates coming from processed white flour or processed white sugar, you're putting strain on your pancreas. And even if it's not a fetal pancreas, it's so easy to switch to cookies made with a whole grain flour, which is denser, more consistent, and actually tastes of the earth. Unfortunately, they're hard to find in supermarkets.

- **White sugar, brown sugar, or sucrose**. Note that the color—brown, for instance—makes no difference on its nutritional value. Remember: sugar is a nutritional void.

  * **All candy, hard or soft.** Candies are primarily made of sugar, along with added color and flavoring, inviting one and all to indulge.

* **Sugary soft drinks.** This type of beverage consists mainly of two things: water and sugar. More than half have over 100 grams of sugar per liter; that's the equivalent of 20 sugar cubes. You might remember New York City mayor Michael Bloomberg imposing a ban on soda cups over half a liter in volume a few years ago. Bloomberg was actually aware of my work fighting invasive sugars and asked for my support for his project. It was a happy day for both of us when the city's health department authorized the ban. Unfortunately, the American Beverage Association succeeded in pressuring the federal government to reject the measure.

* **Sugary sorbets and ice cream.** They consist of fruit juices to which sugar and water are added. Ice cream is more caloric than sorbet because it contains milk or eggs, which is to say proteins and lipids that slow down the penetration of sugar. During these two months, resolutely set aside the sorbet and avoid ice cream if possible.

• **Noodles made from soft wheat.** These should be left on grocery store shelves until your baby's pancreas is more mature. It's not much to ask. Other kinds of pasta are easy to find. Spaghetti, cooked *al dente*, for example.

• **Dates**. These are probably the most sugary fruit that has ever existed. Dates and raisins are the only dried fruits that you should really avoid altogether during these 60 days.

List II: High-carbohydrate foods to AVOID during the crucial two months.

The first list contained foods that you should *eliminate* because they are too aggressive for your unborn child. The second list contains foods you should *avoid,* in descending order.

For this second carbohydrate list, what matters most is the notion of quantity. If you're a perfectionist and you're able to totally avoid the products it contains, I commend you—I think that's the best strategy. But if you and your doctor think you can consume those foods occasionally, be very sure to limit the quantity.

- **Standard white rice.** This is the kind you get in Chinese or Japanese restaurants. If you can't avoid it, try to leave some at the bottom of the bowl. And, remember to avoid sticky rice, which is white but more invasive; it's on the list of foods to eliminate.

- **Finely ground white couscous.** Couscous comes in three sizes: large, medium, and small. The smallest version is the one to avoid. Couscous is further proof of the fact that the more you physically or chemically process a food, the less work is required during digestion, the less resistance the food meets, and the more quickly it arrives in the blood.

  The large size couscous—essentially, Moroccan Berber couscous—is almost impossible to find and takes a few minutes more to cook. If you like a grainy consistency, you'll love this kind.

  Whatever the size, avoid cooking this grain for long. This accelerates the transformation of carbohydrates into glucose.

- **Ordinary semolina.** For these two months, choose whole grain semolina.

- **Bread with 30 percent rye.** Specifically, this is bread *with* rye, containing 30 percent of that ingredient, and not *rye bread*, which has about 60 percent rye. The difference between the two kinds is that the 30 percent difference usually consists of white flour.

- **Canned corn.** The kernels stripped from the ear have aged in the can and are steeped in liquid; they're predigested, robbing you of the opportunity to do the digesting.

- **Ice cream**. You'll notice that I made a distinction between ice cream, which is to be avoided, and sorbet, which is to be eliminated. That's because ice cream, while having more calories, contains milk, cream, or eggs which slow down carbohydrate absorption.

This distinction should highlight the fact that calories matter less than the categories they belong to. It might seem like splitting hairs, but it's one of the main reasons the fight against excess weight and diabetes is so often thwarted. For a long time now, a concerted effort has been made to hide the dangers of invasive carbohydrates. One of the most effective tactics is to claim that "one calorie = one calorie" and that "all calories are equal."

This apparently simple, logical idea belies a monstrous deception, conscious or otherwise. The unit of measurement casts a veil over *what it is* we're measuring. Think of it like this: if 1 gram really equals 1 gram, 1 gram of cyanide is equal to 1 gram of baking soda.

The same goes for the popular and longstanding myth that proteins are harmful to the kidney. This is simply a smokescreen to make us forget that it's sugar, not proteins, that are responsible for damaging the kidneys.

Similarly, Coca-Cola recently focused its marketing on physical activity, skillfully leading us to think that if you increase your level of physical activity, you can keep drinking sugary sodas.

- **Ripe bananas**. Bananas are already one of the most high-glycemic fruits. As a banana ripens, the starch chains transform into infinitely more invasive glucose, meaning its glycemic index level rises even higher. The same phenomenon takes place when you cook a banana, and for the same reasons.

- **Cooked beans**. Why not try them raw, young, and tender, without the shell? In this form, you can indulge to your heart's desire.

- **Buckwheat flour**. Aside from its high amounts of carbohydrates (72 grams/100 grams), buckwheat is allergenic. According to Dr. Castelain-Hacquet, head of allergology at France's Saint-Vincent de Paul hospital, "there were 14 cases of severe anaphylaxis to buckwheat since 2010, including five in 2014. All the patients treated received a first aid kit containing adrenalin." If you love buckwheat pancakes, wait until your pregnancy is over.

- **Canned pineapple**. Pineapple is a fruit that's high on the glycemic index, and eating it canned in syrup bumps it up even higher. You may have heard that the fruit contains bromelain, a magic enzyme that melts cellulite. This is a myth. This enzyme facilitates the digestion of proteins, but not fats, and especially not cellulite.

- **Well-cooked white spaghetti**. In the third list, you'll see that spaghetti cooked *al dente* is tolerable, but the same pasta cooked for longer is not, for the small developing pancreas. I'll risk becoming repetitive here and say it again: the more extensively a food is processed, the faster you will absorb it, and the more negatively it will impact your own and your unborn child's pancreas. Cooking is part of that transformation. If a diabetic could eat raw potatoes, there would be no reason to prohibit them, but in their ready-to-use flaked form, it would be dangerous.

- **Regular ketchup**. Ketchup is a mixture of tomatoes, vinegar, and sugar. Its carbohydrate level is 26 grams/100 grams. A fresh tomato contains only 3.9 grams, and mustard has 5 grams. Try making your own ketchup. If you have time, start with fresh tomatoes; if not, use tomato paste.

- **Well-cooked bulgur**. The same is true of pasta made from hard wheat. Excessive cooking heightens its invasive power.

- **Long-grain brown rice and red Thai rice**. These are less invasive than white rice, but you should still avoid them during these crucial 60 days.

- **Nutella**. You'll probably be surprised to find Nutella in the category of foods that are to be avoided and not eliminated outright. The reason for this is that the fat content that accompanies the sugar slows its progression.

- **Whole wheat bread**. This, too, is to be avoided. The word "whole" is misleading. All it means is that wheat has been added to white flour. Beer poured into a wine glass is still beer.

- **Whole wheat pasta**. To be avoided for the crucial two months. On the next list, you'll see that you can eat whole grain pasta, cooked *al dente*.

- **Sweet potato**. It's better than regular potato, but still, wait for two months.

- **Prepackaged pizza**. Avoid this because of the flour. After the crucial two months are over, make your own pizza with whole grain flour—and don't forget a spoonful of olive oil to slow down the sugars.

- **Basmati rice** (long grain). If you love the flavor of basmati, there is an acceptable whole grain version in List III.

- **Honey**. This should really be avoided during those two months. Even though it's a natural product, it's adapted for bees, not humans, and especially not for a developing fetus. Honey is a near-pure mixture of fructose and glucose.

- **Canned lychee**. This is to be avoided.

- **Waffles**. Avoid store-bought waffles; they're made mainly with white flour. But, if you want to take the time to prepare whole grain or oat bran flour yourself, that's an option.

List III: Foods tolerated in moderate quantities.

The third list doesn't contain foods to eliminate or even to avoid. These are foods you can consume. But that doesn't mean you should overdo it. Don't forget what you've learned earlier in this chapter on how to calculate the glycemic load. The point isn't for you to be an expert in the nutritional information that diabetics need to know. The main thing *you* need to know is that when it comes to carbohydrates, quality is as important as quantity.

Thus, this third list contains foods that you can eat, but not in excessive portions. Warning: while these foods have an acceptable quantity of sugars, they can still accumulate and reach unacceptable levels very quickly.

- **Wild rice**. This would be your best option for rice—if it were actually rice. Wild rice is an aquatic plant that's hard to find. Overcooking it can make it unappealing. The best solution is to let it soak in water for a few hours or overnight before cooking.

- **Whole grain basmati rice**. Even though it's Indian in origin, eat it Italian style: *al dente*.

- **Tabbouleh**. Enjoy this Lebanese style, with lots of parsley, mint, onions, and tomatoes mixed in with the bulgur.

- **Bulgur**. A type of cracked wheat that's shelled and precooked.

- **Vegetable wheat**. Vegetable wheat differs slightly from bulgur because it is whole and not crushed.

- **Store-bought tomato sauce**. It does contain sugar, but in reasonable amounts. If you want to, you can find sugar-free sauces as well.

- **Pumpernickel**. A heavy German bread rich in fibers and minimally processed grains.

- **60% rye bread**. Not *with rye* but *rye*—an important distinction.

- **Whole grain couscous.**

- **Whole grain kamut and kamut bread**. This is a species of wheat whose grains are quite a bit bigger and harder than ordinary wheat, which gives it a more resistant husk. It is also slower to break down and lower on the glycemic index. Unfortunately, you may only be able to find it in health food stores.

- **Whole grain wheat flour**. Stone-ground flour that is minimally sifted; it isn't stripped of its bran, germ, or starch.

- **Whole grain spaghetti or other whole grain pasta, cooked *al dente***. Add some butter and Parmesan to slow the absorption of carbohydrates.

- **Sugar-free whole grain breadsticks**. Don't forget that these tolerated foods add up in combination.

- **100% whole grain sourdough.**

- **Raw cider**. To give you some idea:

  * 5 fluid ounces of raw cider = 1 cube of sugar

  * 5 fluid ounces of sweet cider = 2 cubes of sugar

  * 3.4 fluid ounces of Madeira wine = 2 cubes of sugar

  * 8.5 fluid ounces of beer = 2.5 cubes of sugar

* 3.4 fluid ounces of Muscat dessert wine = 4 cubes of sugar

- **Coconut milk**. A jewel for cooks who want to give their dishes an exotic touch and a richer flavor. It's a main ingredient in Thai food and part of the reason the cuisine is so popular today. For those who might be tempted to eat too much of it, you can cut the amount and mix equal parts coconut water. It's also a great milk replacement for those who are lactose intolerant.

- **Agave syrup and coconut sugar**. If you're reluctant to use sweeteners that are totally carbohydrate-free, these two natural sweeteners are good substitutes with low glycemic effect.

- **Pumpkin and squash**. Both are great to eat in soups during the crucial 60 days.

List IV: Carbohydrates to eat freely.

The fourth list contains foods that are high in carbohydrates but whose molecular configuration makes them slower to digest and absorb, and therefore less disturbing for your baby's development. As you will see, this book's enemy isn't carbohydrates, but rather, their penetrating power.

The tolerated foods mentioned in this list cover the vast majority of your pregnancy needs—as well as your gustatory pleasure—but without placing violent demands on the pancreas of the beloved little passenger in your womb. As you select and prepare your food, don't forget that everything you put in your mouth will be shared with him or her.

Remember that all the carbohydrates you ingest become glucose. Glucose generates insulin, and insulin is the cause of the problems we're concerned with. So, if you eat a club sandwich on white bread, or a plate of risotto with a beer, massive amounts of glucose will flood your blood and your child's blood. This unexpected concentration of glucose requires the fetus to produce insulin, and also to create new endocrine beta factories to produce that insulin.

Our objective during this period is to help you get the carbohydrates you need, bit by bit rather than in avalanche form, to avoid the brutal spike in blood sugar and the massive release of insulin from your pancreas. Be like a mouse walking quietly in front of a sleeping cat, trying not to wake it. During those two months, choose "silent" foods.

So, what are these silent carbohydrates? They are foods on this list; those you can eat normally, without worrying.

- **Peas and chickpeas**. These are the champions of slow carbohydrates. Prepared properly, they can make great replacements for starchy or floury foods.

- **Kidney beans, black beans, yellow or brown lentils**. These are food powerhouses: dense, filling, rich in fiber, and high in nutritional value.

- **Stew and homemade sauerkraut**. Avoid canned foods.

- **Nectarines**. Try not to have more than three portions of fruits per day during the crucial 60 days.

- **Rye crispbreads**. These are made of up of 24 percent fiber.

- **Apples, oranges, pears, grapefruit, currants, cherries**. Remember: three portions a day will suffice.

- **Fresh tomatoes.**

- **Tomato juice**. Tomatoes have high nutritional value, and their lycopene content helps prevent certain cancers.

- **Sugar-free tomato sauce**. These can be store-bought or homemade.

- **Quinoa**. A trendy food that's rich in proteins (16 to 18 percent) and iron, high in biological value, and free of gluten. The grain has a caviar-like texture that bursts when you bite it, with a slight hazelnut flavor. It's great in savory and sweet dishes alike.

- **Yogurt and white cream cheese/cottage cheese**. These are sugar-free, but not necessarily light.

- **Sugar-free diet chocolate bar**.

- **Green beans**.

- **Artichokes**.

- **Dark chocolate, 70% or higher**. In moderation, if your doctor is monitoring your weight. The sugar in the chocolate is slowed by the accompanying fat.

List V: Recommended carbohydrates.

The last list contains virtuous foods: those that you're not only permitted but encouraged to eat, especially if you have an active lifestyle.

Neuroscientists know that at every level on the animal scale, habit is a kind of biological impulse that promotes individual safety and survival. Any behavior that is repeated and doesn't lead to harm is recognized as safe and is admitted. But if a behavior proves more than merely safe and ends up gratifying and soothing, it is installed in our brain circuitry as a desirable habit.

Pregnancy is generally one of the most rewarding events in a woman's life. The habits that develop during that time take deeper roots than most. So, to make your pregnancy as safe as possible, take up the habit of reducing your consumption of invasive carbohydrates.

It'll be that much easier to keep the habit going after you give birth, especially if you have weight problems or a family history of diabetes, cardiovascular disease, or cancer.

Here the very beneficial foods you can eat on a daily basis.

- **All vegetables**. Choose, in particular, all kinds of cabbage, zucchini, mushrooms, any type of lettuce, cucumber, radishes, leeks, spinach, peppers, fennel, endives, tomatoes, and eggplant.

- **Lemon, strawberries, and raspberries**.

- **Hearts of palm**.

- **Snow peas**.

- **Oilseeds**. These include nuts, hazelnuts, almonds, pine nuts, avocados, and olives.

- **Rhubarb**. This is tart, rich in fibers, and extremely low in carbohydrates. Try making compote, fresh-tasting and rich in fiber. The icing on the cake is that rhubarb is rich in antioxidant polyphenols, and it was recently discovered to contain parietin, a pigment that can inhibit the growth of cancerous tumors.

- **Lupin flour**. You can use this as an addition if you are preparing pastry. Its glycemic index is as low as that of oat bran.

- **Cacao with 1 percent fat**. In recent years, cacao has been available with lower and lower amounts of fat: first 21 percent, then 11 percent, and finally 1 percent. Try the latter. It's great for baking and gives you that slightly euphoric chocolate feeling so many of us love.

- **Oat bran**. This is a food I truly love. Its primary virtue is that it can perfectly replace flour for almost any usage, without compromising its incredible glycemic index level. It's extremely useful to keep the following in mind:

While glucose has a glycemic index of 100 (think about it as the maximum speed of a car), white sugar and sucrose have a glycemic index of 70, and today's white flour has a glycemic index of 80, the glycemic index of oat bran is 15.

These are the elements you should respect for those crucial days that are so important for the future of your pregnancy. As you can see, the recommendations are clear, simple, and easy to follow.

During these essential two months, you can eat anything that is healthy and beneficial. You won't be missing anything you need, and you won't be consuming processed invasive carbohydrates. Those foods are dangerous for adults in the medium term, if they consume them regularly and with abandon. And if they're dangerous for adults, they're even more so for a developing baby—especially during those 60 days when the power to synthesize insulin starts to form.

Months 6, 7, 8, and 9 of Your Pregnancy

Over the last four months of your pregnancy, the developing pancreas becomes mature and functional, and starts secreting insulin. If the expectant mother hasn't been careful with her diet and (like most of us) has consumed more invasive sugars than the pancreas is prepared to deal with, the child she carries will enter the sixth month with a pancreas that is already enlarged and secreting insulin before schedule.

If the diet remains the same during these last four months, the unborn child will continue to secret insulin and to gain weight as a result. As this situation occurs, other parameters come into play, such as maternal weight and personal or family propensity for diabetes.

If the expectant mother began the pregnancy overweight or obese, or if she has a history of insulin resistance, she's at risk of developing gestational diabetes and causing her child to be born with a birth weight higher than 7.7 pounds.

But, if she has carefully controlled her consumption of invasive sugars:

• Her child will have a healthy pancreas.

• She herself will have gained the appropriate amount of weight—normally between 22 and 29 pounds.

• She will not be at higher risk for gestational diabetes.

• Her child won't be vulnerable to excess weight or insulin resistance, nor to metabolic syndrome or diabetes.

Starting from the sixth month, the cells of the pancreas (now a properly formed organ) multiply less, but grow larger. The little pancreas follows the development of these cells, becoming larger and producing more and more insulin until birth.

During the same period, the mother's body naturally goes through a period of insulin resistance. This is perfectly natural. This helps her to gain weight, improving her chances of carrying the pregnancy to term. The process is inscribed in our genetic score. However, the danger today is actually abundance, rather than lack; that means you need to be very aware of this natural tendency. The intensity of the insulin resistance varies according to maternal body weight before pregnancy, the number of previous pregnancies, and family history of excess weight or diabetes. Here, again, the remedy is the same:

master your blood glucose by limiting the foods that raise it too high, too often.

In the last trimester, all your body's cells, especially those of the liver and muscles, will lose some of their sensitivity to insulin. That means you'll need more insulin to neutralize and suppress the same quantity of glucose. If your diet remains too rich in invasive carbohydrates, you therefore run the risk of damaging your pancreas. It's usually in the dietary and hormonal context of the third semester that weight gain starts to get out of control and the risk of gestational diabetes increases.

The dietary guidelines intended to protect the fetus during this last phase of pregnancy will benefit you if you're at risk of gestational diabetes. Today, there's some debate about increasing monitoring for gestational diabetes, especially for at-risk women. Risk level is related to the presence of excess weight, a family history of diabetes, and previously giving birth to a large baby. Gestational diabetes may be unpreventable in some cases. If it does appear, reducing sugars is not enough, and insulin is needed.

That means that limiting invasive diabetogenic sugars in order to protect the fetus can also benefit the mother: both pancreases face the same threat.

During the last four months of pregnancy, it's wise to stick to Your Daily Diet in Five Basic Steps (page 91). These principles are enough to constitute a solid line of defense for the fetal pancreas.

But these rules go beyond protecting your child. With practice, they can become dietary reflexes that will protect you from the artificial and diabetogenic diet that we've come to think of as normal. Its recent invasion directly correlates with the global epidemic in excess weight, obesity, and diabetes.

Therefore, it's a good idea to continue this food plan past your pregnancy, to integrate it into your daily life, and to share it with the people you care about. Foods as common as corn flakes, instant potatoes, sugary sodas, and white bread are not foods for humans. Why? Because we have neither the organs nor the physiologies to assimilate them safely.

For the last two months of your pregnancy:

- Follow the crucial 60 days' list of foods to eliminate: List I: High-carbohydrate foods to *eliminate* during months four and five.

- Follow the crucial 60 days' list of foods to avoid: List II: High-carbohydrate foods to *avoid* during the crucial two months.

- You may eat from the following list freely (however, try not to exceed three portions of fruits per day): List III: Foods tolerated in moderate quantities.

- You can eat normally, without worrying, the foods on the following list, which contains foods that are high in carbohydrates that are slower to digest and absorb, making them less disturbing for your baby's development: List IV: Carbohydrates to eat freely.

- Eat more of these foods every day: List V: Recommended carbohydrates.

Conclusion

As you come to the end of this book, I hope you have been persuaded to follow the plan for the crucial 60 days of your pregnancy.

If you're starting a pregnancy and you *haven't* been convinced, you still have three months to reflect—three months in which your child's pancreas does not yet exist. Consider carefully: a diet low in industrially processed foods is simply a return to the diet your grandmother had when she was carrying your mother.

So much evidence exists today on how harmful invasive sugars are for an adult human that it's easy to ignore the effect it can have on the little being inside you.

On the other hand, if you've decided to follow the plan, then nothing could make me happier. And in that case, I'd like to ask for your help in taking the plan further.

How? Merely by keeping a simple journal of your diet for the six months of the plan.

There are two reasons I'm asking you to do this.

One, it will be a way to collect and keep information on your consumption of carbohydrates over the most important 60 days of your pregnancy. It can then be analyzed in combination with all the other journals, and used to fight weight and health problems in the children born of these pregnancies. The more readers who send in their results, the more meaningful the results will be.

Today, we know that the obesity and diabetes epidemic manifests very early on. One of the first warning signs is birth weight. Even more important is the weight of the infant at six months, and more important still is the weight at two years.

To make it easy for you, I created a website at www.baby6months .com so you can monitor the development of your pregnancy. When you visit the website, you can open your own personal account. Your account will have weekly calendar, from the ninth to the thirty-ninth week. During the fourth and fifth months, each day of the week contains two lists, one with foods to eliminate and one with foods to avoid.

Each day, click on the foods you've consumed from these two lists to show if you've eaten a little, a moderate amount, or a lot, so the results can be tabulated. It only takes a few seconds.

At the end of your pregnancy, enter the gender, weight, and birthday of your child. And if you're willing, also enter your child's weight at six months, one year, and two years. If enough data is entered, it will help prove (or disprove) the fundamental point that is the basis for this whole project.

And if the basis of this book is proven correct—and I'm certain it will be—imagine the satisfaction of knowing how much you've done for your child's health and future. And imagine my satisfaction at having helped you get there.

Conclusion

If you follow the plan in this book, I invite you to write to me with any questions you might have throughout your pregnancy. This book is being published in about 20 languages simultaneously, and I may receive a fair number of questions—so if you can, try to keep your questions within the scope of this project.

In closing this book, I'd like to wish you the best for the journey of your pregnancy. I have two kids myself, and the powerful joy, energy, and happiness of the event of their births is something I carry with me every day.

As a child, I lost my beloved grandmother when she fell into a diabetic coma and passed away a few hours later. I've distrusted sugar ever since, and I only consume it in very moderate amounts. My wife feels the same.

So, without knowing the epigenetic explanation underlying it, my wife's diet during her pregnancies was fairly close to what I have recommended in this book. What's more, back then (my eldest child was born 33 years ago), industrial food hadn't reached the intense degree of transformation of today's foods. My children were born with a normal weight, and they have no problem controlling their weight today.

My deep love for my family inspires me to protect them, which is why I mention them here, and I know that the same motivation is guiding you. The plan in this book takes that motivation a step further: It aims to make your pregnancy, and every pregnancy, a healthy one. Through this plan, we share a common goal. Thank you for joining me. I'll support you every step of the way.

References

Barlow, D. P., R. Stoger, B. G. Herrmann, et al. "The Mouse Insulin-like Growth Factor Type 2 Receptor Is Imprinted and Closely Linked to the Tme Locus." *Nature* 349, no. 6304 (January 1991): 84–7.

Bourc'his, D., G. L. Xu, C. S. Lin, et al. "Dnmt3L and the Establishment of Maternal Genomic Imprints." *Science* 294, no. 5551 (December 2001): 2536–9.

Cattanach, B. M., C. V. Beechey, and J. Peters. "Interactions between Imprinting Effects in the Mouse." *Genetics* 168, no. 1 (September 2004): 397–413.

Cattanach, B. M., and M. Kirk. "Differential Activity of Maternally and Paternally Derived Chromosome Regions in Mice." *Nature* 315, no. 6019 (June 1985): 496–8.

DeChiara, T. M., A. Efstratiadis, and E. J. Robertson. "A Growth Deficiency Phenotype in Heterozygous Mice Carrying an Insulin-like Growth Factor II Gene Disrupted by Gene Targeting." *Nature* 345, no. 6270 (May 1990): 78–80.

Drewell, R. A., J. D. Brenton, J. F. Ainscough, et al. "Deletion of a Silencer Element Disrupts H19 Imprinting Independently of a DNA Methylation Epigenetic Switch." *Development* 127 (2000): 3419–28.

Gosden, R., J. Trasler, D. Lucifero, and M. Faddy. Rare Congenital Disorders, "Imprinted Genes, and Assisted Reproductive Technology." *Rapid Review* 361, no. 9373 (June 2003): 1975–77.

Harding, Anne. "Downing diet soda tied to risk of premature birth." Reuters. July 23, 2010. http://www.reuters.com/article /us-diet-soda-idUSTRE66M4AF20100723

Hark, A. T., C. J. Schoenherr, D. J. Katz, et al. "CTCF Mediates Methylation-Sensitive Enhancer-Blocking Activity at the H19/lgf2 Locus." *Nature* 405, no. 6785 (May 2000): 486–9.

Hata, K., M. Okano, H. Lei, et al. "Dnmt3L Cooperates with the Dnmt3 Family of de Novo DNA Methyltransferases to "'Establish Maternal Imprints in Mice.'" *Development* 129, no. 8 (April 2002): 1983–93.

Kono, T., Y. Obata, Q. Wu, et al. "Birth of Parthenogenetic Mice that Can Develop to Adulthood." *Nature* 428 (April 2004): 860–4.

Landers, M., D. L. Bancescu, E. Le Meur, et al. "Regulation of the Large (Approximately 1000 kb) Imprinted Murine Ube3a Antisense Transcript by Alternative Exons Upstream of Snurf/ Snrpn." *Nucleic Acids Research* 32, no. 11 (June 2004): 3480–92.

Lee, M. P., M. R. DeBaun, K. Mitsuya, et al. "Loss of Imprinting of a Paternally Expressed Transcript, with Antisense Orientation to KVLQT1, Occurs Frequently in Beckwith-Wiedemann Syndrome and Is Independent of Insulin-Like Growth Factor II Imprinting." *PNAS* 96, no. 9 (April 1999): 5203–8.

Lewis, A., K. Mitsuya, D. Umlauf, et al. "Imprinting on Distal Chromosome 7 in the Placenta Involves Repressive Histone Methylation Independent of DNA Methylation." *Nature Genetics* 36, no. 12 (December 2004): 1291–5.

Li, E. "Chromatin Modification and Epigenetic Reprogramming in Mammalian Development." *Nature Reviews Genetics* 3, no. 9 (September 2002): 662–73.

Li, E., T. H. Bestor, and R. Jaenisch. "Targeted Mutation of the DNA Methyltransferase Gene Results in Embryonic Lethality." *Cell* 69, no. 6 (June 1992): 915–26.

Lopes, S., A. Lewis, P. Hajkova, et al. "Epigenetic Modifications in an Imprinting Cluster Are Controlled By a Hierarchy of DMRs Suggesting Long-Range Chromatin Interactions." *Human Molecular Genetics* 12, no. 3 (February 2003): 295–305.

Lucifero, D., M. R. Mann, M. S. Bartolomei, et al. "Gene-Specific Timing and Epigenetic Memory in Oocyte Imprinting." *Human Molecular Genetics* 13, no. 8 (April 2004): 839–49.

Mager, J., N. D. Montgomery, F. P. de Villena, et al. "Genome Imprinting Regulated by the Mouse Polycomb Group Protein Eed." *Nature Genetics* 33, no. 4 (March 2003): 502–7.

McGrath, J., and D. Solter. "Completion of Mouse Embryogenesis Requires Both the Maternal and Paternal Genomes." *Cell* 37, no. 1 (May 1984): 179–83.

Obata, Y., T. Kaneko-Ishino, T. Koide, et al. "Disruption of Primary Imprinting During Oocyte Growth Leads to the Modified Expression of Imprinted Genes during Embryogenesis." *Development* 125 (1998): 1553–60.

Reece, A., G. Leguizamón, and A. Wiznitzer. "Gestational Diabetes: The Need for a Common Ground." *Lancet* 373, no. 9677 (May 2009): 1789–97.

Reik, W., W. Dean, and J. Walter. "Epigenetic Reprogramming in Mammalian Development." *Science* 293, no. 5532 (August 2001): 1089–93.

Rougeulle, C., C. Cardoso, M. Fontes, et al. "An Imprinted Antisense RNA Overlaps UBE3A and a Second Maternally Expressed Transcript." *Nature Genetics* 19, no. 1 (May 1998): 15–6.

Rougeulle, C., and E. Heard. "Antisense RNA in Imprinting: Spreading Silence through Air." *Trends in Genetics* 18, no. 9 (September 2002): 434–7.

Sleutels, F., R. Zwart, and D. P. Barlow. "The Non-Coding Air RNA Is Required for Silencing Autosomal Imprinted Genes." *Nature* 415, no. 6873 (February 2002): 810–3.

Surani, M. A., S. Barton, and M. Norris. "Development of Reconstituted Mouse Eggs Suggests Imprinting of the Genome during Gametogenesis." *Nature* 308 (April 1984): 548–50.

Thakur, N., V. K. Tiwari, H. Thomassin, et al. "An Antisense RNA Regulates the Bidirectional Silencing Property of the Kcnq1 Imprinting Control Region." *Molecular Cellular Biology* 24 (September 2004): 7855–62.

Umlauf, D., Y. Goto, R. Cao, et al. "Imprinting along the Kcnq1 Domain on Mouse Chromosome 7 Involves Repressive Histone Methylation and Recruitment of Polycomb Group Complexes." *Nature Genetics* 36, no. 12 (December 2004): 1296–300.

References

Verona, R. I., M. R. Mann, and M. S. Bartolomei. "Genomic Imprinting: Intricacies of Epigenetic Regulation in Clusters." *Annual Review of Cell and Developmental Biology* 19 (2003): 237–59.

Wutz, A., O.W. Smrzka, N. Schweifer, et al. "Imprinted Expression of the Igf2r Gene Depends on an Intronic CpG Island." *Nature* 389, no. 6652 (October 1997): 745–9.

Index

About the Author

Pierre Dukan is a French doctor and nutritionist who created a totally new method for perceiving calories and diet. In 2000, after 30 years of experience in working face-to-face with patients, he decided to publish his life's work, The Dukan Diet. The book quickly became a bestseller and has been translated in over 26 languages. He is also the author of 19 other books. Many stars and celebrities swear by his nutrition program.

Faced with the global inability to control the epidemic of overweight and diabetes, Dukan attacks the issue in this new book: at the root, in the mother's womb, at the crucial moment when the mother's diet plays a major role in the development of the baby's pancreas.